The
ANXIETY
COACH

Michael Hawton, MAPS, is a registered psychologist and a former school teacher. He has worked in the area of child and family psychology for over 30 years. He has published two previous books on child behaviour management, both of which have been translated into simple Chinese. Michael has prepared many hundreds of child protection and family court reports. He has been employed as a consultant in population-change projects by UNICEF. For the past 17 years, he has specialized in training family educators, school leaders, teachers and parents in behaviour management. Michael's practical approach equips children and young people with the skills to manage their emotional over-reactions. A father of two, Michael brings a clear, no-nonsense approach to managing anxiety in children and tweens.

The
ANXIETY
COACH

Every parent's guide to building resilience in their child

MICHAEL HAWTON

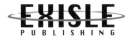
EXISLE
PUBLISHING

First published 2023

Exisle Publishing Pty Ltd
PO Box 864, Chatswood, NSW 2057, Australia
226 High Street, Dunedin, 9016, New Zealand
www.exislepublishing.com

A CiP record for this book is available from the National Library of Australia.

ISBN 978-1-922539-58-8

Designed by Enni Tuomisalo
Typeset in PT Serif, 11pt
Printed in China

This book uses paper sourced under ISO 14001 guidelines from well-managed forests and other controlled sources.

10 9 8 7 6 5 4 3 2 1

Disclaimer
This book is a general guide only and should never be a substitute for the skill, knowledge and experience of a qualified medical professional dealing with the facts, circumstances and symptoms of a particular case. While this book is intended as a general information resource and all care has been taken in compiling the contents, neither the author nor the publisher and their distributors can be held responsible for any loss, claim or action that may arise from reliance on the information contained in this book. As each person and situation is unique, it is the responsibility of the reader to consult a qualified professional regarding their personal care.

Praise for *The Anxiety Coach*

'In a time where we are seeing more young people struggle with anxiety, Michael Hawton's book comes powering to the fore with encouragement and practical strategies for parents to get their child's anxiety back under control. As a GP, I see an increasing number of parents seeking help to cope with child anxiety with limited access to psychological services.'

— Dr Ann Staughton

'*The Anxiety Coach* details how parents can help prevent children catastrophizing the inevitable challenges of "growing up" and reminds us all to enjoy the journey.'

— Dr Martin Whitely, PhD., author of *Over-prescribing Madness*

'As a paediatrician, I often see children with anxiety and parents want to know what they can do to help their child. This book provides a much needed, easy to use resource for parents to understand and manage their child's anxiety.'

— Dr Fiona Noble MBBS FRACP, paediatrician

'More children than ever before are experiencing anxiety. This is a great resource and an easy read for parents. *The Anxiety Coach* provides realistic examples and exercises for parents to empower their child to manage their anxiety and develop resilience.'

— Kathie P. Mackay, pre-school director

'This book is a common-sense approach to parenting anxious children. It gives real-world examples and techniques for helping children negotiate uncomfortable situations; allowing them to blossom, rather than to hide.'

— Vanessa, teacher and mother of two

Contents

Part 3: The Anxiety Coach tactics

Preface

After a long career as a community psychologist and talking with parents about their children's behaviour problems, I can draw a distinction between an earlier time and now. In the 1990s, I saw a lot of parents who complained that their children were answering them back or just not listening. These were the main reasons that parents came to see me. In other words, most parents were having problems with their children's *behaviour*. At one stage, I had a six-month waitlist for a first appointment in my practice. Back then, I estimate that over 80 per cent of my caseload was seeing the parents of children with difficult behaviour. The remaining 20 per cent of my client load involved children who were anxious. Nowadays, things have changed. I can safely say, more children are behaving anxiously compared with previously.

So, is it possible that we are seeing more and more children affected by anxiety? Or are more people perceiving situations as more anxiety-provoking than used to be the case? Some childhood behaviours don't seem that serious at first, and often parents think children will grow out of certain problematic behaviour. However, without the right intervention, anxious behaviour can often escalate over time.

One way anxiety manifests in children is in the development of faulty thinking habits. A child's anxiety can manifest itself in the form of anxious talking and anxious behaviour. Anxious 'talking' can be heard when a child overuses words or phrases like, 'I'm stressed' or 'I can't cope'. Anxious 'behaviour' can be noticed when we see a child being more reticent or more wary than usual. Often, when children with anxiety concerns are not doing well, they tend to avoid situations they find uncomfortable, unless they have learnt how to overcome their anxious feelings or fears. Overcoming these anxieties is something that can and must be learnt by children as they weigh up how to respond to life's difficult moments. It's also something you are in the driver's seat in supporting them to do. Helping your child be the boss of their anxiety will be one of the most important parenting tasks you will ever undertake.

You'll want to encourage your child to be brave, to take risks and to try out new things — but the problem is that if you're short on time or you don't want any drama, there's always a temptation to jump in to 'fix' things or to take charge of the situation where you end up solving problems *for* them. Children are naturally on the lookout for their parents' help so they can cope. Most parents are reluctant to simply witness their child's distress. When this happens some of us give in to our child's reticence. This type of parent behaviour is very common. But there's a middle path between backing off and challenging your child to face their fears, which is what I want to show you.

I will show you how to help your child not freak out at the whiff of a problem, and that's what we'll be focusing on: how you can help your child handle life's problems, constructively.

The main process I will show you in *The Anxiety Coach* is one in which *you* will play a starring role in helping your child develop capacity to handle life's challenges. The plain truth is that if your child is to be the boss of their anxiety, you will need to teach them how to do it. It doesn't come naturally. If you can imagine a future situation where your child was emotionally stronger and you only had to a do a minimum amount of calming maintenance of their mental state, that's what I would like for you.

In the book I give a guide for helping your child manage anxiety in the preschool to the thirteen-year-old age group. I give you:

  » case studies from families and children I have met

  » a flowchart to help you make quick decisions

  » a few simple worksheets to complete, and

  » tips for implementing what's in the book.

What the book is about

There is now broad agreement among anxiety researchers that about one-third of anxiety in children is due to genes and temperament, while two-thirds of anxiety habits are learnt. This means that children mostly *learn* anxious thinking habits in the way they interact with others or situations.[1] Even if your child is temperamentally predisposed to anxious behaviour, you will be able to show them the necessary skills for managing their anxious behaviour once you have read this book.

Dealing with your child's anxiety is going to take time. You will need to know how to respond when your child says or does things that indicate they may be feeling anxious. Anxious behaviour is often an interplay between a child's environment, thoughts and feelings. A parent can learn 'serve and return conversations', which will enable a child to engage with stressors and learn to moderate their feelings. As we will see, the development of a strong 'sense of self' in children is formed through exchanges between the child and responsive adults — including parents, educators and other significant adults. As children move into middle and late childhood, their peers, social media and their wider social context will increasingly influence their sense of identity and belonging.

When a child enters a situation that provokes some worry or anxiety, a parent can respond in a way that reduces the likelihood the child will develop anxiety. If a child is experiencing an anxious moment, these exchanges between the child and their carers can either exacerbate the child's anxiety or help the child form a healthy brain architecture. If the child has too little of the right type of interaction, the likelihood they will become more anxious increases. By contrast, alternative types of interaction will help a child to forge a resilient mindset — one that can manage everyday stresses. The actions you take in that micro-moment (something I call 'the short game') matter, and if you repeat these positive exchanges over and over (something I call 'the long game') you will build your child's lasting resilience.

From the beginning, I want to draw the distinction between a child who behaves anxiously and a child who is diagnosed with an anxiety *disorder*.[2] All people, including children, experience some anxiety at some points in their lives. All children worry about certain things like whether their mother or father will always be around or whether their friend really likes them. But anxiety is on a continuum. At the extreme end there are anxiety disorders, which affect only about 7 per cent of children. Not all children with anxiety progress to an anxiety disorder. A key difference between the two is that if a child has a disorder, their anxiety may prevent them from doing normal activities that are part of being a child, like going to school, socializing with friends or engaging with challenging but otherwise normal activities (e.g. going for a bike ride or going with family on a holiday).

The average age a child is diagnosed with an anxiety disorder is eleven years old.[3] By intervening early when you see your child displaying fretting behaviour or other anxious behaviour, you can help your child learn to manage their thoughts and feelings and practise coping strategies. Wherever your child is on that trajectory, there are ways to intervene and build a path to great resilience.

What you can achieve with this book

Parents and carers can be instrumental in making a difference to how a child manages their anxiety. By reading this book, you're off to a good start.

That said, it's not unusual for parents to delay seeking help for a child's anxiety, because they might think their child will grow out of it. It's also common for parents to wonder who they might get the right help from to address a child's anxious behaviour. Still other parents are 'put off' by the expense or long waitlists they might encounter if they try to seek professional help for their child. Furthermore, general counselling is not the preferred treatment for a child with anxiety because the evidence does not support its effectiveness. For children who have an anxiety disorder, professional help should be undertaken with someone who specializes in teaching cognitive behavioural strategies to children.

While these days it can be tempting to think you might need to rely on first-tier professionals like a GP or a psychologist to remedy a child's anxiousness, you don't have to. With the 'right' training, there is little difference in treatment outcomes for children if they see a psychologist or a parent if they are coached by a parent.[4] Using the strategies outlined in this book will be less costly and, unlike going to see a psychologist (who, at best, might see your child for six to eight sessions of therapy and achieve significant results) you're the one there on the ground with your child. As such, you will more readily see and hear opportunities throughout any one day when you can use the practices in this book to help your child overcome their worries.

Relatively modest changes in how you and other significant adults respond to your child's anxiety can make a significant difference to whether your child exhibits anxiety symptoms. These changes are broadly known as family management strategies.[5] Even if you learn relatively few of these strategies, you can help your child become less anxious. You can use the techniques I will show you to also ward off any serious anxious behaviour in the future. These day-to-day exchanges with your child will help them to stop and focus on how they can manage stress.

If you notice your child is speaking or behaving anxiously, it is important to take stock of what is happening and work out whether to step in. The biggest factor preventing parents taking action is their lack of confidence in making a difference to their child's anxiety. We don't want to do the wrong thing, or we think this is the domain of mental health professionals. If this is your experience then I suggest you read on, because once you muster the confidence that you're doing the 'right thing' your behaviour will be more consistent and purposeful. Your child's life is going to be full of ups and downs and you will need to prepare them for the best and worst that life will serve up. We can't protect them all the time. So, as the saying goes, better to 'prepare the child for the road, not the road for the child'.

I propose a 'less of/more of' model of intervening in your child's anxious behaviour. The 'less of' part of the book involves you doing some things less often to reduce your child's anxiety. The 'more of' part of the model (in the later sections of the book) involves you being proactive in developing your child's ability to manage their anxiety. You can coach your child in the skills they need to learn to develop their emotional strength. Just as non-emotional skills are learnt (such as learning how to eat with a knife and fork) so, too, can emotional skills be learnt (such as knowing how to cope with worry or fear). My goal is to give you the confidence to know what to say and do in given moments when your child is anxious. To some extent, these actions by you will need to become automatic. Your life is probably busy enough, so if I offer quick-fire ways for you to act — a form of decision hygiene — these actions will become easy enough for you to implement in the right moment.

I'll introduce you to the SALON script for holding conversations with your child in an anxious moment. This script will give you a 'go-to' response to use in most instances of anxiety. SALON stands for:

» **s**elf-check first, and come to a 'full stop'

» **a**cknowledge how your child is feeling

» **l**ist what you have noticed and make the invisible visible

» ask **o**pen-ended questions

» **n**ow what?

You can use the SALON script as a routine way of responding to your child's anxiety. If you repeat all or even some parts of it, it will help your child think like a scientist, to assess what's going on, to learn to question anxious thoughts and feelings and to work out a way forward. You need not wait for their school to show them how to think like a scientist. It is possible for even preschool children to learn a scientific way of looking at the world and how to manage their own anxieties.

In the final section of the book I will give you an anxiety-conversation cheat sheet. If you like, you can put this on your fridge door as a memory jogger.

How the book is organized

Part 1 (chapters 1 to 5) investigates **knowledge** about how anxiety operates — **and how its opposite, resilience, works**. If you can get your head around some simple understandings of how children develop a strong, healthy 'sense of self', you can use the right parenting tool at the right moment to fix anxious habits when you observe them. Nothing too abstract, as far as theory goes. But I will provide you with enough information to enable you to understand what's happening in anyone's brain, especially your child's! By having a more objective grasp of anxiety and how it operates, you can make this new understanding work in your favour.

Part 2 (chapters 6 and 7) looks at how patterns become established in families — and how to change them. A pattern of behaviour in a family takes a bit of time to form and, as far as children forming anxious habits is concerned, it's important to know how some very common patterns in families are set up. We'll learn this because when you're conscious of how a pattern becomes established, it is possible to change that pattern. The skills I will teach you will help you not just become aware of patterns and how they function in all families, but also how to change a pattern.

Part 3 (chapters 8 to 12) looks at proven techniques used by mental health professionals to change anxious behaviour in families. There are key techniques I will unpack that are each aimed at the same outcome: helping your child to develop emotional strength so that even when you're not there, they can apply the skills you've shown them, at times when they are feeling anxious. I will give you a worked example of how to use SALON, when you notice your child speaking or behaving anxiously. I will also ask you to work out an action plan for implementing what you have learnt in the book with your family.

Imagine if you taught your child a skill (such as how to interrupt their anxious thinking) and you saw them using that same skill without you having to prompt them. Wouldn't this be a wonderful thing to see? You'd see the lightbulb go on in their ability to take control of their anxiety and you would be the person responsible for making it happen.

The skills you'll learn will make a lot more sense if you can see a family applying the skills in their home.

Meet the Coopers

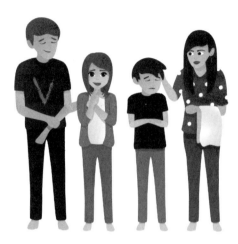

This is Jane and Andrew Cooper and their two children.

Jane is a 36-year-old mum who works four days a week as an account manager at a construction company. Andrew is a 39-year-old dad and is a local pharmacist. Their children are Emma, eleven years old, and Tom, eight.

Let's look at how the Coopers have approached anxiety issues in their family using some of the strategies for change we'll be looking at in Part 3 of the book.

In recent months, the Coopers have found themselves ...

- trying to distract or placate Emma when she becomes emotionally heightened and fretting
- reassuring Tom when he pesters his mother to ensure she will 'be there' to pick him up from tutoring

- finishing off (or actually doing) Emma's schoolwork when she hits a snag in her completion of a school task
- giving in to Tom's avoidance of going to school
- changing what they do at home (e.g. not eating out) because Emma doesn't want to.

Given the way things have been going, Jane and Andrew could see the writing on the wall. They recognized that if they kept doing the same things over and over, as in the above examples, they would become increasingly annoyed at having to fit around their kids' anxiousness (adjusting how they normally behaved as a family). They also saw that their children were becoming pernickety about what they would and would not do.

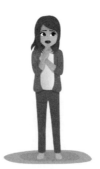

Emma is a flamboyant child who tends to create problems for herself and her parents by becoming fixated on the smallest frustration. Lately, Emma tends to emotionally heighten when she is asked to fit in with some family boundaries, such as getting off her phone or sitting with the family for dinner.

She's been refusing to eat out with her family because she doesn't like using other people's cutlery. Emma is also a perfectionist. Whatever she does she must get it right — or else she just won't attempt to do it. She excludes herself from many things for fear of not getting it right. She'll lockdown onto a hard 'no' if something doesn't *feel* right. Emma consistently wants her mother to check her homework. In class, she is reluctant to present her work to the teacher or to put up her hand. Her parents have seen her burst into tears over what they assess to be challenging, yet largely manageable, tasks. Their concern is that Emma appears 'fragile' and she 'falls apart' when faced with seemingly small challenges.

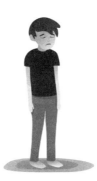

Tom is slightly less anxious than his sister. But he has one main problem. He lets out his nervousness by seeking reassurance and checking that many things will be done by his parents. Tom is also often worried about fitting in. He probably worries too much about what other kids, or his teachers, think about him. Lately, Tom has been reluctant to return to school. When he has a socially awkward day at school (with his friends) he'll want to stay home the next day. In other words, he avoids anything with a whiff of friendship difficulties. Recently, he has been having more days off than days when he goes to school. He has been pestering his mother for constant reassurance that she will pick him up from after-school tutoring on time.

Throughout this book, we will delve into how Jane and Andrew typically respond to their children's anxiety but also how they replace what they 'normally' do with more productive ways to support and challenge their children.

The table on pages 16–17, which we will fill in throughout the book, shows the types of behaviour Jane and Andrew have developed in reaction to Tom and Emma's anxious behaviours. Their consciences are pricked every time they find themselves behaving this way. Part of them wants to be sensitive to how their children are feeling, while another part of them knows it is not good for either their children or themselves if they acquiesce. I will identify what a child learns from sub-optimal decision-making, and in Part 3 I will introduce five replacement actions Jane and Andrew can use to respond to their children's anxious behaviours. As we move through this book, I will complete the other columns: what the child learns from a parent behaving like this, and what you can do instead.

To begin with, let's look at the structure of this book. It is based on three strong foundations. They include:

» how to help a child keep things in proportion

» how to help your child not be swayed by external events when solving problems

» how to help a child rely on their mind rather than being over-influenced by external factors, such as what others think or a prevailing fashion.

There are so many people telling parents what they should be doing. I suppose I am one more voice among the cacophony of opinions! That said, I learnt a thing or two by being a teacher on how to simplify ideas and put these ideas into a meaningful sequence so that they're not complicated for the learner. The other aspect of this book I hope you will find useful is that I will be very clear in what I say to you. I'll give you evidence-based processes for helping your child to overcome anxieties they may face in the future. If anything, I'm hoping to give you clarity and purpose as you read the pages.

Let's get started.

Actions by parents

Signs of anxious behaviour	What the child says or does	What parents might normally do
Emma 'feels' distressed in her body and becomes fretful, frantic or volatile.	'I can't do that! No, no I can't just "feel" this way.' (She reels from the event/situation.)	Jane placates, distracts or gives in to Emma. Becomes exasperated.
Tom pesters his mother to ensure she's going to 'be there'.	Tom keeps asking, 'Are you sure you'll be there?'	Jane keeps reassuring Tom, saying, 'Yes, I'll be there.'
Emma invites Jane to do her school project.	Emma says, 'Can you do it for me?' (When Jane doesn't, Emma gets more upset.)	Jane might normally jump in to fix things. She doesn't want to risk a drama and ends up doing the task for Emma.
Tom 'avoids' friendship problems by not going to school.	Tom 'locks down' quickly on a 'no'. He forms a habit of catastrophizing.	Andrew helps Tom avoid a challenging situation by letting him stay home.
Emma doesn't want to go to places or do normal family things. Her bandwidth of 'normal' narrows.	Emma avoids participating in normal tasks. She wants her parents to agree not to do certain things.	Jane and Andrew 'accommodate' by changing a family routine e.g. not eating out at restaurants.

What the child learns from the parents' reaction	Teach the child a coping micro-skill instead

PART 1

The anxiety scene

Child anxiety has become endemic in western societies. In the next five chapters, we will explore key information about why anxiety has developed into such a major issue facing children. You'll learn the main factors that have contributed to this steady rise in child anxiety over time. You'll also learn about what parents might be tempted to do when faced with their child's anxiety, and how to allow your child to take some risks within their capacity to manage.

1.

Foundational ideas

A parent's job

Our first foundational idea is to define what a parent's job is. For most jobs, a company works out ahead of time the role description for the person their job advertisement is trying to attract. If I was to hazard a guess at a *parent's* job role, I'd say it boils down to one main thing: to help their child reach maturity. Part of growing up is developing the ability to control our strong feelings. One writer who has attempted to define what it is to 'grow up' is a psychiatrist called Dr Scott Peck. In the 1970s, Peck wrote a book called *The Road Less Travelled*, in which he described that, as we mature, we develop a certain capacity to balance our emotions in proportion to the events we face.[1]

> » If someone looks at me the wrong way, just how much should I let that sour face make me feel sad?
> » If I don't get an invite to my friend's party, just how much should I let this event affect my mood?
> » If I don't like the teacher, just how much should I let my dislike for this particular teacher affect my motivation to go to class?

In the greater scheme of things, any of these events may be a 4 out of 10 event — and probably deserve a 4 out of 10 reaction. Depending on how we see it, though, it might evoke an 8 out of 10 reaction in us. A different event, such as a threat to a member of your family, may be a 9 out of 10 event that triggers a 9 out of 10 reaction — a level of reaction that might be entirely appropriate according to Peck's view on maturity.

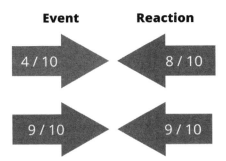

Children experience their own anxieties but because their brains are still developing, they interpret events differently.

What children interpret as worrying will be different to what *we* experience as adults — not just because they are a different person to us, but also because they are at a different stage in their development; that is, their experiences are subject to certain cognitive limitations. It's not that they're less intelligent, but rather it's more that their brains are still growing.

Working out what is worth worrying about can be tricky if you're a child. Clearly, not every situation is a 9 out of 10 event. However, in children who become overly anxious we might see a disproportionate reaction to something you might consider not worth worrying about. They haven't yet learnt how to gain control over their anxiety. Children's ability to harness their feelings depends partly on the stage of development they are at (meaning we would expect them to develop greater ability as they move onto another stage) and partly on learning and practising the skills they need so that they can manage their worries and concerns (meaning that with the right help they can use those skills to 'return to calm').

Locus of control

The second foundational idea is to consider how we want our children to solve life's problems. To explore this, I want to talk with you about a concept called locus of control — a concept first developed by Julian Rotter in the 1960s.[2] A child's locus of control is their future problem-solving orientation. Does your child think that *others* determine their ability to solve problems, or do they see these problems as being largely within their control? For example, some children believe that the *causes* of their feelings come from external factors or that luck or chance is more in charge of them than they are of themselves. This can be a problem as far as anxiety goes. If you believe that your anxiety is caused by others — and cannot be sorted out by yourself — this can limit your ability to manage anxiety. If you have an external locus of control, you can end up believing that your feelings are the result of what happens *to you*. So, in your assessment of what is making you anxious, you prefer to see external circumstances as causing your anxious feelings. Children are necessarily more externally oriented and with the right training can be helped to become more internally oriented.

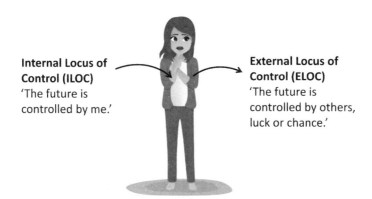

Internal Locus of Control (ILOC)
'The future is controlled by me.'

External Locus of Control (ELOC)
'The future is controlled by others, luck or chance.'

According to Rotter, a child's locus of control can be located on a continuum, with one end being an internal locus of control and the other end being an external locus of control. 'Internals' believe it is important that they take steps on their own behalf to solve problems in an 'I can do it' approach to life. When I left university in the 1980s roughly 50 per cent of people had an internal locus of control and 50 per cent had an external locus of control. When my university lecturers talked about this concept, they didn't put a value judgment on it. They didn't say whether or not one end of the continuum was associated with good or bad outcomes. The thing is, they would now!

A recent meta-study (a study of 43 different studies) showed that for around the last 50 years there has been a steady increase in the number of people who say that their orientation is located externally.[3] In other words, more people say that many things in their lives are not in their control. Today, children are 80 per cent more likely to be 'externals', and 'externals' don't fare as well as 'internals'. Eileen Ahlin's work in this space is also seminal. She says externals do less well academically and are just more anxious.[4]

Some people ask if locus of control is a personality issue. In other words, they're asking if this is something that is fixed or if it can be changed. The answer to that question is that a child's locus of control is mostly learnt and, importantly, it can be shifted from an 'external' orientation to an 'internal' orientation with the right help and coaching.

There are two important things to know about a child's locus of control. The significant adults in a child's life (including teachers) can influence their locus of control, and the development of an *internal* locus of control orientation has long-term benefits for your child's wellbeing. This is excellent news because significant adults can do many things to generate an internal locus of control in children — even in very young children. In a parent-led model, you can orientate yourself and how you respond towards your child developing an internal locus of control way of thinking — with all the benefits that that brings. You've just got to know what to concentrate on, and then keep practising that skillset to build your child's internal locus of control.

The triangle of wellbeing

A third and final piece of our foundational ideas puzzle is how we work out how to calm or soothe ourselves as we grow older. Daniel Siegel uses a simple diagram to explain how this works. In his 'Triangle of Wellbeing' model, he first shows us that, as an adult, we can use our mind to calm our nervous system.[5] We might go for a walk at the end of the day to decompress the day's events or write a list of pros and cons to consider a problem, or talk things out with a friend.

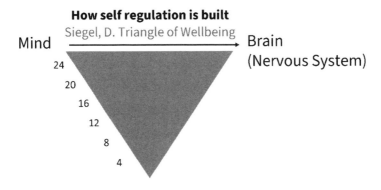

Adults can self-soothe. It's not that we don't need our relationships with others, but we are more independent in working things out the older we become. An adult might also find ways to stop themselves from worrying, by interrupting their cycling thoughts or calming down their body by doing some breathing exercises. An adult's mind is much more resourceful and able to return to equilibrium under their own steam. An adult might interpret an event as being more tolerable than they first thought. This, and many other skills, come with having an adult mind. In other words, as an adult, we can use our medial prefrontal cortex area (located in the front of our heads, just behind our forehead) to 'tell' the rest of our nervous system to cool it or to get a grip! It's only when a person reaches full maturity — in their early twenties — that they have optimized this capacity for self-soothing.

Until then, young children need an adult to help them to return to calm.

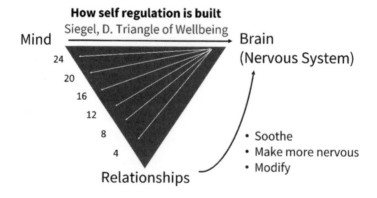

How self regulation is built
Siegel, D. Triangle of Wellbeing

Mind — Brain (Nervous System)

24
20
16
12
8
4

Relationships

• Soothe
• Make more nervous
• Modify

At four years of age, children are much more dependent on their relationships to help them settle after a distressing event. Just as parents and those caring for children can cause a child to feel nervous by behaving erratically or being abusive, they can also help a child to modify their emotions and 'wrestle' with their anxiousness. A parental hug or consoling words are obvious ways that parents can achieve this outcome.

While they are young, children use a less sophisticated lens to look at the world, one that is more emotional than it is reasoned. Young children experience emotions more in their body than their mind. Unlike an adult who can use their mind to return to calm, a child will need a parent to scaffold their ability to modify their fears. And, as we will see, as they get older, not only do their fledgling abilities to manage their thoughts and feelings improve but they can also sort out the things that are really worth worrying about, versus those that are not.

A central task in *The Anxiety Coach* is for me to provide you with strategies to support your child to modify any anxious reactions they might have. However, to do this will involve you at times being comfortable with your child being *uncomfortable*. It will help them to develop healthy brain architecture. I'll have more to say about this in coming chapters, but this is what teachers do every day; they 'stretch' the child's ability by challenging them to do a task that may be just outside their comfort zone. This is a facilitating role, not a reassuring one. Too much reassuring, as it turns out, can have a negative effect on a child in developing their internal locus of control. You might find this surprising. It's not that we will never want to console a child. Of course, you will — and you should. You will express empathy and support and give them a hug when they need one. However, you will also help your child to become an ace problem-solver who gets in the habit of looking at the facts and who looks at alternative ways of seeing a problem.

In the next chapter, we'll look at the opposite of anxious thinking — and how we can help a child to become emotionally stronger. If you can strive towards helping your child to be emotionally stronger, you can effectively kill two birds with one stone: reducing your child's anxiety while simultaneously building up their emotional reserves so they can handle life's future problems.

Summary

» A parent's job is to help a child get things in proportion. Most events are not 9 out of 10 events.

» A child with an external locus of control will do less well at school and is more likely to experience anxiety. Locus of control is malleable, meaning that it is possible to shift a child's orientation from external to internal through family management strategies.

» A child gets better at self-soothing as they get older. But, at a young age, a child is more dependent on the adults around them to learn the processes by which they can modify their anxious reactions.

2.

Definitions of resilience and your role in promoting it

I imagine you wouldn't want to stifle your child's personality in any way. But you will want them to be happy and strong. And I imagine you would want your child to be resilient.

Some people call resilience the ability to 'bounce back'. Others define it as the capacity to maintain one's purpose and integrity in the face of changed circumstances. Here is my favourite definition, by psychologist Rick Hanson: 'Resilience is like the keel of a sailboat; it keeps you balanced and moving forwards.'[1] The boat might be pushed over or put off course every now and then, but over time it will self-correct. In Hanson's sailboat analogy, the craft is robust and sturdy. It has been designed to withstand forces that would otherwise tip it over and throw it off course. The keel keeps the craft 'weighted' in the water while it travels through time.

Unfortunately, I haven't come across many clearly defined methods for how to develop resilience in children. For all the talk about resilience, it's hard to find the right resources to build it. You might well ask, is it possible for a child to become stronger through their exposure to adversity? The answer is yes. A way of thinking about resilience is that it can only develop in real-world circumstances. That is, by facing difficulties in real-time we can help a child develop skills 'on the job'. And, having survived that skirmish, they will take that experience with them into their future encounters with adverse events.

Emergency services professionals often hone their skills by doing simulations of events or disasters. By being as close as possible to real-life situations, they can work out solutions they wouldn't have otherwise thought of.

Nassim Nicholas Taleb is a professor of risk economics at New York University, and he might have some answers for us. He says that children should *not* be protected from all painful emotional experiences. Taleb says *some* things get stronger when put under pressure.[2] They are the opposite of fragile. There are no words to describe the opposite of fragile, so Taleb refers to something that gets stronger through dealing with adversity as 'anti-fragile'. For example, bones need to be placed under regular pressure to maintain their strength. Children who get the measles vaccine receive a bit of the virus so that they develop antibodies — making them less susceptible to getting a more serious illness. Some things need to interact with stressors so that they can grow and develop. Taleb uses the notion of hormesis — a word coined by pharmacologists to denote a situation where a small dose of an otherwise harmful substance can be beneficial for the organism, acting as a medicine.

As far as resilience is concerned, we would hope children get better at developing anti-fragile skills if they get help to manage stresses and problems. Being anti-fragile is an important component of being resilient. In this book, we'll pursue the idea that 'resilience' or 'anti-fragile' thinking skills are *constructible*. And your child will need as near to real-life opportunities as possible to develop these skills. I've heard people use the term 'crucible moments' to describe times when, under pressure, they had to come up with solutions.

Resilience is constructible

An analogy that works in regard to constructing resilience is that of rendering. When plasterers render something, they apply layer upon layer of plaster. With each additional layer, the structure gets stronger.

By helping children develop narrative structures that err on the side of thinking accurately and proportionally, we can also help them think in healthy ways. If we can help children to navigate difficult moments — helping them to thread together different coping narratives — they'll become mentally stronger. More reasonable, rational mental discourses can be laid down experience by experience and solution by solution. By equipping them with adaptive processes, we're in a sense hardening their mental strength.

The Center on the Developing Child at Harvard University has recently distilled decades of research to come up with four essential ingredients that go into helping a child develop resilience.[3] They are:

1. A child needs at least one stable, caring and supportive relationship between themselves and the important adults in their life.

2. Children need to develop age-appropriate *mastery* over their life circumstances. Those who believe they have some measure of control over their lives tend to do better. Simple things like mastering how to make your own bed go a long way towards a feeling of being in control of your life.

3. Children need to develop strong executive functioning and self-regulation skills.

4. Children do better if they are part of an affirming faith or cultural tradition.

These personal characteristics are developed over time. They can be built and developed in a child through having difficult experiences and in subsequently overcoming them.

Driverless cars are a good example of something that gets better with experience. The way it works is this: autonomous vehicles go on to the road with a few basic operations — a first draft, if you will. They 'know' to stop at red lights and keep away from the kerb. With different experiences, autonomous cars become more sophisticated through a process called 'machine learning'. They accumulate more skills (such as how to avoid a car coming towards them) as a result of using pre-existing information that they store in their computer memory. I'm sure you'd agree it is kind of weird that a machine can learn! But the point is that they learn different things from different experiences — and consequently, they adapt. They need those experiences so that they can improve.

For children to develop resilience they need numerous opportunities to make sense of life stresses. They need experiences of struggling followed by the satisfaction of having successfully coped. By having repeated opportunities to take risks and overcome those risks, they will have successfully wrestled with their anxiety. They will then be able to generalize what they learn to future adverse events. Your children will probably find it hard to begin with — there's no getting around that. But you can help them to develop the right processes to become more resilient.

How do you teach resilience?

To become proficient at anything requires practise — lots of it. All the books on sports success say much the same thing: that to become proficient at your game, you first of all need to learn from a good coach, take their feedback (something called 'corrective feedback') and then practise, practise, practise. Getting corrective feedback is important.

Most sports stars had to start somewhere. For any sportsperson to succeed, it takes long-term commitment and drive. Let's take one of the world's most famous sportspeople, tennis player Ash Barty. In the beginning, she had to learn the micro-skills (how to hit the ball, how to use her backhand, how to serve properly). Then, through repetition, by doing drills and through a series of trial-and-error situations — along with corrective feedback — she became proficient. After a while, she became versatile on different parts of the court. She developed a variety of skills that saw her eventually become a world champion.

I like to say Ash Barty was both coached and was coachable. Initially, her coaches knew more about the game, and how it was played, than she did. They may not have been as talented as she was, but they had certain skills and qualities she did not. They were her teachers; they coached her and gave her pep talks. For Ash Barty, no doubt she had to have the right disposition towards her training — and she would have wanted to succeed. She had to be open to being coached. She had to embrace that there would be setbacks. But, above all, she had to have a *willingness* to be trained.

You see where I'm going with all this, don't you? You can be your child's anti-fragile thinking coach! My job is to teach *you* the micro-skills you need to train your child in so that you can help them develop their capacity to wrestle with anxious thoughts and feelings. Then, it's over to you to apply those skills throughout your child's life. To instil a resilience mindset in your child requires coaching them in those micro-moments when they experience anxiety and then your repeated expression of their ability to solve problems. If you can be their mentor and teach them what they need to practise, they will cope better each time they face future adversities. In a sense, this new way of approaching things — which some people call developing a mindset — is like teaching your child a new language. It'll involve learning to ask the same questions a scientist would ask: what's the data? Where's the evidence for my thoughts and what alternative explanations are there? But I am getting ahead of myself. In later chapters, I will show you how you can help your child get into the habit of interrogating their thoughts and feelings with a view to lessening their anxiety.

Believe in yourself

To put *your* best foot forward in helping to reduce your child's anxiety it's very important for you to embrace the idea that you generally know more than your child as far as these kinds of things are concerned. Even before reading this book that was the case. For starters, you have a fully adult psychological mind. They don't. You're also the one reading this book. They aren't. You're the one learning about what can be done to alleviate your child's anxious habits. This isn't an elitist thing to say. It's just a fact that you have had more experience with the ups and downs of life than they have. And, given your age, you have had more experiences in pulling yourself together than they have had.

Some parents suffer from self-doubt about their role and about imposing too much of their influence on their children. They may secretly ask themselves, 'Who am I to influence my child one way or another?' In psychology, this is known as imposter syndrome. It's where you think you are not in any position to be coaching anyone else to do something. It's where you either don't feel worthy or capable enough to do something that's up to you. In exploring a parent-led approach for reducing anxiety, I want to instil confidence in you that you can be your child's lead trainer. This skillset can be taught by you, coached by you — and practised by you in your day-to-day interactions with your child.

Another one of my aims is to give you the skillset you'll need so that you can help your child become as proficient as possible at managing their stress. This is what I call the 'short game' — teaching a small set of modest skills (truly, they are not that hard) and then repeating those modest skills over time. Your goal in training your child is so that they can ultimately independently manage their anxious feelings. This is not a form of therapy such as a psychologist or GP would provide. Rather, it's an orientation by you over the medium term. You can still be the happy-go-lucky parent. And you can still be the caring and loving parent who is compassionate and indulging. It's just that you can be the guide and the coach at other times, too.

Ash Barty only became a better player after years of coaching and training. Just as Barty received, your child will also need corrective feedback. When the coach is in coaching mode they are most interested in teaching the skill involved — and so they are focused on being *objective*. If you are to become good at being the coach, you will need to become an 'objective observer' of your child's reactiveness rather than being too affected by their distress. You need to remember, it's not about you and how you might feel; it's about you teaching them a skill in the micro-moment. As your child's coach, you would expect them to listen and not muck around. Even if the player looks a little impatient or uncomfortable, the coach will keep going. At times, the coach might need to remind or prompt the player to pay attention. Sounds challenging, doesn't it? Well, it is, at one level. I'll have more to say about a parent feeling a bit 'icky' while being a child's coach in later chapters.

Coming up, I will describe how you can anchor your efforts to help your child by applying one theory for improving their emotional control. If you have even one theory, it will give you a way of doing things that will not only provide you with a solid basis for your own behaviour, it will also make things simpler. You just need to follow the theory!

There are so many situations available to you in which you can coach your child for their long-term benefit. Every time you apply an internal locus of control solution, you are building their resilience. If you think about this task as helping your child to develop a series of mental blueprints for straight thinking, you'll be on the right track! At times your help will be in the form of being a 'supportive presence' while they are in the middle of facing a problem. At other times, you will be teaching them 'offline' about how to manage fears or insecurities.

Summary

» You can help your child develop emotional strength, but they need real-world practice at overcoming adversity.
» It is possible to construct resilience.
» While there will be improvements in a child's ability to understand things because of their increasing development, you will need to help them learn how to limit their anxiety.

3.

Some theory needs to drive what you do

Parenting is more complicated than it used to be. After a long stint as a parent and as a psychologist, I have a little perspective about what's changed in the world of parents. Some of these changes include many more parents wanting to get it 'right', almost to the point of perfection compared with parents of a previous generation. What comes with this aspiration is a sense that we're also more sensitive to implied criticism. And then there's the image-sharing: I am now seeing so many more parents having to live up to the image of being the perfect family 24/7! And if I was given a dollar for the number of times I have heard a parent say, 'I just want my child to be happy', I'd be a rich man. There's one more thing: the current-day atmosphere for parents is much more affected by others' judgments. I'm seeing more parents feeling judged.

In these kinds of situations, a simple theory can really help to make things less complicated when you're not sure what to do. It can also give you something to focus on if you're lacking in confidence. If you can go with a theory in a critical moment of your child's anxiety, you will be less dependent on your feelings. I am not saying that feelings are not important; they can be. What I am saying is that feelings are an *unreliable* barometer for our assessment of what's going on. If you rely only on your 'feelings' to guide you, chances are that you will be inconsistent or erratic in what you say and do. For children who need consistency (and that is most children by the way), this can represent unpredictability.

All of us will have days when we're not feeling on top of things. If you have one strong 'theory' beacon to set your course by — in relation to treating your child's anxious habits — this will guide you on those days. If you don't have a theory, you might end up being affected by how *you* have been parented (often unconsciously), which might be good, but not always.

Daniel Goleman says that for children to learn how to emotionally self-regulate they need to do three tasks: identify emotions, track emotions, and then manage their emotions. And it's a hierarchy; you can't do the final task without the first two tasks having been accomplished. Another one of my favourite authors in the resilience field is a psychologist called Joan Rosenberg. She says that children first monitor emotions, then modulate emotions in order to modify emotions.

Children can be taught to *modify* an emotional reaction to an event. But to do that, they first have to monitor and modulate emotions — and again, it's a hierarchy, you see. You can't do the last step without having done the first two steps.

Case study: Travis

Twelve-year-old Travis (and his mother) was the subject of a report I was once asked to prepare for a court hearing to determine if he should be returned into his mother's care. My task was to interview Travis to assess his ability to self-regulate.

It was clear from reading the documents in his case file that Travis had behaved quite violently. I learnt that Travis had been in the child protection system for the previous five years. During that time, he had been suspended from school multiple times, had been violent towards his mother, towards his teachers and towards a school principal. Consequently, there were three apprehended violence orders in place against him. Travis had been diagnosed with oppositional defiance disorder and autism. When I met Travis, I came to the part in my interview where I wanted to talk with him about a recent altercation he'd had with his teacher. He had exploded in a rage and assaulted his teacher. Here's how the interview went.

Me: So, Travis, I was reading in this report [I point to one of the report documents in Travis's view] that you hit your teacher a couple of weeks ago. I want to talk to you about that. Where did it happen and how did it start?

Travis: In the classroom. The teacher wanted to take my iPad off me.

Me: How did you feel about that?

Travis: I didn't want her to take it.

Me: Okay. So, you didn't want her to take your iPad. I hear you saying that. But I didn't ask you that; I want to know how you *felt* about her wanting you to take your iPad.

Travis: I dunno.

Me: [I look at Travis and said something a bit provocative] Travis, did you feel happy?

[Travis spits at me.]

Travis: Don't be stupid! I didn't feel happy!

Me: Okay, so tell me how you felt. I want to know *how you felt*.

Travis: [Travis scrunches up his face, snarls at me] I got annoyed, okay!

Me: Cool, alright. So, what happened next?

Travis: The teacher kept coming towards me; she wanted to take my iPad off me. I didn't want to give it to her.

Me: Okay … how did you feel then?

Travis: [He looks at me quizzically again, scrunches up his face and blurts out] This is stupid! Why are we doing this?!

Me: [I lean in a bit more, lower my voice — with a slight grizzle — and look him in the eye] Well, I'm interested to know how you *felt*.

Travis: [Travis looks down and his face shows he is very uncomfortable.] I told you I didn't want her to take it!

Me: I get that. I do. But tell me how you were feeling at this point.

Travis: [scrunches up his face] I don't know. I got mad!

Me: So, you went from being annoyed to getting mad … and then?

Travis: She shouldn't have tried to take it!

> **Me:** I get it — you didn't want her to take it. But what did you feel next?
>
> **Travis:** She made me 'really' angry.
>
> **Me:** You went from being annoyed to mad to being angry — and then what happened then?
>
> **Travis:** Awww! I just lost it then. That's what I always do!

All of this might appear to any outsider like pulling teeth. However, *the process* I was using was part of my assessment to determine whether Travis was able to exert *some* self-control. I wanted to find out if Travis had any ability to find the words to describe his feelings. In my report, it was my job to give the court an opinion about whether Travis could successfully be reinstated to his family, and under what circumstances. One of the issues was to assess if Travis could be rehabilitated so that he would not be as violent.

You see, in this instance, Travis had *some* capacity to identify his emotions — something you will remember Goleman talked about. Rosenberg calls this ability monitoring. Travis wasn't very good at having these feelings and at managing his reactiveness. He hadn't been trained, given his history. This didn't mean that he couldn't get better at it. One of the key things I learnt about Travis was that even though he needed prodding, he was able to identify some feelings. This may seem like a small thing, but it is a first point into my assessment to determine whether he would be able to exercise self-control. He needed training — in the best sense of that word — but he showed some ability to wrestle with his feelings.

Now reflect on *my* behaviour in my conversation with Travis. I want to do this because I want you to think like I was thinking. I am not patting myself on the back here, but you would probably have noticed that I didn't get upset with Travis, even though he was rude and aggressive towards me. It was important for me to remain calm and to lead the conversation in the way that I did, to see if Travis was able to access a 'feeling' language. It did not matter whether Travis liked me and I needed to allow him to not like me, so I could get *him* to do the work.

My assessment process was to ask him questions — ones, as you saw, that made him feel uncomfortable, but which highlighted the limitations in his ability to wrestle with his feeling state. I wasn't doing this to be cruel. Rather, I was 'holding the space' for Travis (neither reassuring him nor backing away from him). I wanted to see if he was capable of tolerating some frustration so that I could make the right recommendations about where Travis should go next, in terms of his rehabilitation. What was missing for Travis, given his family history, was that he didn't have good control — not enough, anyway — to counteract his emotional reactions. In his family, he had learnt from an early age how to argue with his mother. He hadn't been expected to take control of his emotions. You will remember that he said, 'That's what I always do'. This was an indication of a certain rigidity in his response. It implied that he believed he had no alternative but to lose control. Of course, he *did* have an alternative. He could have modified his angry reaction to the teacher's request for his iPad. But the truth is that, at some level, he was making a choice not to.

In much the same way that Taleb talks about how anti-fragile thinking can improve through a series of mini-experiences in managing different situations, so, too, children can gain skills through experiencing some uncomfortable feelings — even painful ones. Travis was not used to holding any painful emotions without acting out. If only someone in Travis's life could have trained him to tolerate some of that discomfort, he could have been helped to manage himself and his emotional outbursts.

One thing I really like about Rosenberg's work is that she says that feelings (both good and bad ones) are *a form of energy*. Energy can take lots of forms. But the type she refers to is the energy in ocean waves. Waves go up to the shoreline. When the energy in the wave diminishes, the wave eventually recedes. This is an important metaphor. Emotions generally don't tend to last more than 90 seconds, she says. But to develop resilience, we need to get used to riding feeling waves and to help our children do the same. And as uncomfortable as it may seem — and despite our tendency to want to 'rescue' them from bad feelings — it is important to help them ride these emotional waves if they are to develop resilience.

In later chapters, I'll show you some of the ways to facilitate these modifying processes in a child. In particular, I'll show you how you can help a child to wrestle with strong emotion — including anxiety — and ultimately (by you holding the space for them) to go about helping them wrestle with their anxiety. For a parent the hard part of this process is seeing your child struggle, grimace or be generally uncomfortable and not be tempted to jump in to save them.

Catch *yourself* from over-reacting

Seeing a child struggle with strong emotions can be painful for any parent to watch. Most people faced with the likes of Travis would probably want to distract him or get angry back at him. Or you might be tempted to try to rationalize with him. It's easy enough to want to jump in to fix the problem or to yell at someone like Travis. It's much harder to not react.

As I've mentioned before, you may be inclined to want to protect your child when they're anxious or to make things better rather than see them suffer. At times your jumping in can be in the form of reassurance if they are anxious. The only problem with too much reassurance or jumping in to fix a problem for any child is that it won't teach them to rely on their own resourcefulness or to develop mastery over their emotional reactions, which is so important in helping children to develop resilience.

Seeing your child in some emotional pain may not be all bad. If you don't jump in, it does not necessarily equate with a lack of care or that you're somehow being mean. There are lots of times when a child will go through an adverse event, such as getting an inoculation. It can be hard to watch your child being affected by this pain, but you know that you are doing it in their best interests.

I did that with Travis. You may need to do this with your child if they experience an anxious reaction — 'hold the space' for them to help them learn how to manage their anxiety. Remember, I was not that affected by Travis' grimacing and his lack of comfort in what I was asking him. That said, I'm not his parent. If I *was* his parent, of course, I might have been tempted to rescue him from his discomfort by backing away or getting angry with him. As a parent, you will need to override your compulsion to jump in. To successfully help your child wrestle with their anxiety, you will need to set yourself to the side and say to yourself:

> 66 This is not about me. I know they are feeling uncomfortable. But it is not in their best interests for me to simply reassure them. I need to help them develop their emotional strength, and the best way for them to do that is through them experiencing and then successfully managing their difficult emotional experiences.

In the next chapter you'll learn some of the basics of how anxiety operates. If you can understand some of the basic elements of how anxiety works in our brains, you can help your child wrestle with their anxiousness. They can develop skills to be 'the boss' of their anxiety.

Summary

» Using a theory can help you orientate yourself to support your child to identify, track and manage their emotions.

» By 'holding the space' for Travis, I was able to elicit from him that he had access to some words to describe how he felt. I wasn't trying to be cruel to him; I was trying to assess his potential ability to manage his emotions.

» When faced with this level of hostility it can be tempting to back away. Try to hang in there and try not to be affected by your child's struggling.

4.

Anxiety basics

More than a few moons ago — in 2005, in fact — I was asked by my local junior soccer club to take on the job of coaching the under-twelve girls' team. My own daughter was in the team. I had never played soccer as a child, but I had played rugby, and I knew how to play team sports. As a junior player, I knew my coach knew things I didn't know. I knew about how to keep my position and that the game had certain rules.

As far as soccer went, I did not know the micro-skills involved in playing soccer — let alone how to coach a soccer team. So I undertook basic training to be a coach at 'soccer coaching camp', held over two weekends, and I watched some training films. I was surprised by what I learnt: how to kick a ball properly so it stayed low, and how to stop a ball on the spot so I could control it. I learnt how to head the ball without causing my skull to hurt, and I learnt new rules of the game so I could help the girls use the rules to their advantage. By learning some coaching basics I was a better coach than if I had not attended soccer coaching camp.

In this chapter, I will teach you the basics of anxiety — how it functions in the brain and how it's controlled. While I don't expect that you will study psychology or know how to manage a problem with a child with an anxiety disorder, I *do* want to help you understand some basic principles about how anxiety works in a child's brain so that you can be your child's 'brain' coach. You never know, it might also help you to manage any anxiety you may experience.

Stress is not the same as anxiety

One of the first things I learnt in Psychology 101 at university was that stress affects everyone. The things that stress us are called 'stressors'. While everyone faces stressors, some people handle them more smoothly than others. Some events strike up bodily reactions in us. We feel scared or even panicked. Our hearts jump a beat and cause us to rear away from the thing that appears dangerous. The same event can affect different people in different ways. Where one person may face a situation and experience an anxious reaction, another person who faces exactly the same situation does not. Since you're reading this book it's likely your child is one of the first kind of people and you'll need to remember that, because it is highly likely given your child's age they might worry about something that you may not. You might be tempted to tell them not to worry about it. However, that might not be the best action to take in a given moment. I will show you how you can respond in those moments to both help your child manage their anxiety there and then, and also to get better at managing their anxiety for future stressful moments.

To begin with, there are two specific locations where we experience anxiety in our brains: one where we experience anxious thoughts, and another where we experience fear.

Understanding the brain

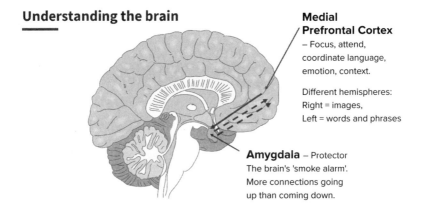

Medial Prefrontal Cortex
– Focus, attend, coordinate language, emotion, context.

Different hemispheres:
Right = images,
Left = words and phrases

Amygdala – Protector
The brain's 'smoke alarm'.
More connections going
up than coming down.

Our thinking brain

The front area of the brain is called the medial prefrontal cortex, otherwise known as our mind. It is the place where most of the brain's neuronal 'wiring' joins up. It's like the cockpit in a plane and controls different parts of the plane. The mind's job is to help us focus, attend to and organize our emotional reactions.

On the left side of that area in the cortex there is a place that uses words and phrases to describe situations. We hope that the words and phrases a child uses will be an accurate reflection of what they experience. But this isn't always the case. If they learn distorted ways of reacting to adversity, then those descriptions can be laid down as incorrect narrative threads in their mind.

Even as adults, our emotional responses to events are not necessarily always well considered ones. But a child can be even more ill-considered at times, because their brain is immature. Children have fewer words to describe inanimate objects, such as things they see in their environment. Children use words like 'one' and 'two' to describe the number of objects they see. They use words like 'red' and 'blue' to denote colours. That's all well and good. But when it comes to naming their feelings, it gets a little more complex. At an emotional level, they might use basic words to describe how they feel: sad, mad or bad. For example, your child might experience worry, and then won't know how to control their worry. They may not yet have learnt enough words or phrases — acting as an inner voice — to look at something from a different angle or to debate with themselves about how much to let a stressor affect them. They'll get there, but it will take a while.

Cognitive distortions

The thing is, even in adults, the left side of the cortex gets things wrong. These distortions are then repeated in a person's mind as the go-to words and phrases they use when facing a challenge, and they can contribute to the development of anxiety. In children, these ways of thinking can become habitual and, if they do, that is when we say a child has developed an anxiety problem. These labels are called cognitive distortions. Cognitive distortions are not good and can make us very unhappy! This is where our mind — having misinterpreted something over and over — ends up *believing it*. The way we describe things becomes what we believe! These are the narrative threads of thought I mentioned before. What we say to ourselves matters. As it turns out, what your child tells themselves about difficult events matters. My wife is a learning support teacher in a high school. She has told me that some boys in her class habitually say to her, 'I'm dumb'. When something becomes too difficult, they blurt out, 'I'm dumb'. How we frame things can be a representation of how we feel, but it is not necessarily an accurate representation of reality.

On other occasions, I've also seen children in my practice who suffer from a form of brain-lock, who have got into a habit of clamping onto default ways of thinking and behaving in much the same way that Travis did (see p. 41). They appear rigid in their responses, unable to tolerate frustration and quite often they are locked into a way of behaving that gets them into trouble. Yet other children let their initial fear of the unknown situation compel them to lock down onto a hard 'No!'. 'No, I don't want to play backyard cricket.' 'No, I can't do that talk in front of the class.' 'No, I'm not going.'

It doesn't help when things are a bit skewed at a societal level. Our culture can send us messages (including to our children) that are exaggerated and inaccurate. So, it's not hard to see why children and young people are affected by what they hear and see.

Australian psychologist Nick Haslam says terms like depression and anxiety are being used at increasingly lower thresholds and across more situations.[1] This lowering of the bar in the application of mental health labels to describe *ordinary stresses* may also increase the number of people who suffer, because it creates a looping effect: using the incorrect labels can change the behaviour of the person doing the labelling and it becomes a self-fulfilling prophecy. So, if a child gets used to saying, 'I can't do that; I have anxiety', this becomes a self-limiting label, whether or not there is a diagnosis.

Adults who observe a child behaving like this are generally reluctant to challenge the child, because to do so looks like they are second-guessing the child or that they are being insensitive.

When adults don't agree with a child, it's not uncommon for a child to say, 'You don't understand me!' or 'Oooh that hurts.' This kind of slight (which implies you're insensitive) can make any reasonable adult back off. So it's tricky for parents and teachers to know what to do when they are facing a child or tween who has all the right 'lines' worked out to stop anyone from challenging them.

While I appreciate that part of being an older child or teenager is to flirt with being overly dramatic and exaggerating feelings, I don't accept that we should allow emotional reasoning or catastrophizing to be open slather. We don't encourage or allow teenagers to smoke, drink, drive or break the law. The same should be the case with the mental habits we see them developing. We need to help them to think more adaptively — particularly if things are not going well for them. Remember, not everything is a 9 out of 10 event — so not everything is just 'awful', 'traumatic' or 'the end of the world as we know it'. When we use more accurate and proportional language — something we learn to do — we can usually work things out, without becoming overwhelmed.

Let's look at the top five cognitive distortions children can pick up.

» **Emotional reasoning** refers to when we *feel* something is bad and deduce that therefore it must be bad. This is thinking with your feelings. Rather than putting the situation under the microscope, we let our feelings determine how we think. Once a child gets in a negative loop of letting their feelings be the filter through which they interpret events, this can be hard to break out of.

» **Disqualifying the positive** refers to when we let one thing that went wrong in a situation come to the forefront rather than looking at things overall. For example, let's say you're doing a presentation and at the very beginning of the presentation you're a bit nervous. But once you get started you overcome your nerves and the rest of the presentation goes as planned. If you disqualify the positive you might let that false start colour your evaluation of the whole talk.

» **Mind reading** refers to when we assume we 'know' what the other person thinks, without any evidence for that belief. Let's say your friend doesn't ask you to a party; you might think, therefore, that she doesn't like you. You don't know this for sure but you jump to a conclusion as if it is the case.

» **All-or-nothing thinking** is where something is perceived as being all good or all bad — no greys in the middle. With reference to yourself you might think either 'I'm a loser' or 'I'm hopeless'. With reference to a situation, it's 'incredibly bad' or 'a complete waste of time'.

» **Catastrophizing** occurs when dramatic words and phrases are applied to what might be a challenging but largely manageable situation. When children use words like 'It was so terrible' or 'I was so traumatized' to describe a situation, they could be making the situation out to be worse than it really was. If their default is to use such words and phrases, these terms can become a habitual way of dealing with even slightly adverse occasions and these interpretations can become second nature.

Cognitive distortions that are not addressed influence the way children explain difficulties or challenges to themselves. Rather than saying, 'It's just a problem, I can work this one out', people who have developed cognitive distortions default to habitual ways of thinking, which can result in them feeling quite avoidant, reluctant or tentative.

In the medial prefrontal cortex, there are clear ways in which we (both adults and children) encode or store information. Look at it as laying down scripts or threads of language on a circuit board. If the information gets laid down incorrectly — and events are routinely misinterpreted — these incorrect narrative structures can morph into an anxiety problem. Ill-fitting mental discourses are ill-fitting because they are not accurate, let alone rational. Anxious habits tend to build and build. The phrases and words being used set up house in a child's mind. If that happens too many times along a historical trajectory, a child can develop poor thinking habits and even an anxiety disorder. Once our thoughts lay 'tracks' in our mind (think of a well-worn path in the countryside), these can become the default tracks that are used when we are faced with adversity.

As a parallel to the cognitive distortions mentioned above, Martin Seligman says the go-to tracks used by 'anxious' teenagers are threefold: teenagers make things *personal* (e.g. 'It's my fault' or 'I am so ugly'), they make things *permanent* (e.g. 'I am never going to amount to much') or they can make things *pervasive* (e.g. 'All the girls hate me').[2] Seligman says that teenagers who have developed these cognitive distortions will come to believe their self-comments. That's what they know and that's what they think. We will come back to cognitive distortions, and how to combat them, in later chapters.

The other side of the cortex thinks in pictures or images. It sees things! In the right hemisphere of our cortex, we *imagine* things and, again, if we let our imagination 'run riot', we might imagine the worst. We can over-imagine things that haven't happened yet. When I was a child, I can remember my grandmother used to say to me, '*Don't meet trouble halfway, Michael.*' What she meant was, don't over-imagine things that haven't happened yet. Good advice, don't you reckon? What a wise owl my grandmother was.

The frontal areas of the brain can lose their bearings, meaning the cortex can fail to keep things in proportion. It can also 'over-try' in attempting to sort out something. This mental process of going over and over events is called 'cycling' or 'ruminating' — and it is a big problem for some children and young people. Going over and over things for no productive outcome can be distressing. If it's about a future event, we call that worrying.

Your child's alarm system

We're covering anxiety basics in this chapter, so I need to tell you about the other area in the brain where anxiety takes place. I need to tell you about … (cue the sound of a smoke alarm going off) the amygdala! This part of the brain has a habit of shooting first and asking questions later. It has a specific job to protect us when we look like we're in imminent danger. It acts without thinking, because in life some things require us to move quickly away from a threat. In a better-safe-than-sorry way, our amygdala is our in-built protector. It is 'old brain' hardware. When the amygdala 'alarm' gets triggered, it releases a hormone called adrenaline. Our heart rate increases, our pupils dilate, we sweat, and large muscle groups prepare for action. A long time ago it played a more pivotal role in our survival. Back then — when we were more exposed to wild animals or marauding invaders — our 'protector' played an important 'fight or flight' role. It didn't ask for an explanation; it just jumped into action. Some things need to happen now!

The amygdala is located about midway between our ears (there are actually two amygdalae — one in each hemisphere). It can also get triggered when we perceive a strong association with some historical danger, such as if we've been previously bitten by a dog. Like any smoke alarm, it can go off at the wrong time, such as when the toast gets burnt. A good way of thinking about a child's ability to deal with the fear messages they receive from their amygdala is that they only have partial control over these messages and, for the other part, they rely on their attachment system with their parents.

Developmentally, children face a double-whammy in managing amygdala-fear events. First, they have an immature amygdala–mind connection. Second, they don't yet have the skills at hand to calm their amygdala without parental help. Not only does their amygdala tend to go off at the wrong time compared to an adult's amygdala, but they also possess a less sophisticated mind than an adult, and they can't tamp down their fear in the same way. As adults, we might be startled in a specific moment, for example being bowled over by a big wave at the beach. If that happened to you or me, we would recover by using our wits to work out what's going on. We'd pull ourselves together nearly as quickly as we became panicked. The wave has passed and we didn't break any limbs. 'Phew, that was a close one.'

On the other hand, a child might be fearful about something an adult would not be fearful of, like patting a dog. They don't yet have the return-to-calm 'chip' installed in the same way that adults do. We need to distinguish between amygdala-based fear and cortex-based anxiety mainly because where each of these anxieties originates has important implications for the techniques we need to use to manage them. If we know the differences, we can use the right techniques to help a child 'return to calm'.

The other thing to know about the two parts — the amygdala and the cortex — is that they are connected by long-range pathways in the brain called *fasciculi*. There are pathways going down from the cortex to the amygdala and pathways going up from the amygdala to the cortex. These pathways are more established in adults — more hard-wired in, so to speak — which means they can more meaningfully communicate with one another. In children, the top-down pathways are not as developed as they are in adults. So kids can't talk to their fear states as readily. While a child can experience fear, they may not be able to manage their fear by talking to themselves like an adult can. A child has not developed a 'second-person' ability to chat to themselves. Here's what I mean by second-person chat. My friend, Kathie, who is 70, told me she was feeling a bit down. 'You know Michael, I just had to have a good talk to myself. I told myself, "Kathie, you are fortunate. You have healthy kids and grandkids, you don't live on the street and you have money to live on. It's okay, you're alright!"' This is an example of Kathie talking to herself in the second person. She had initial feelings of sadness or low mood — but she jumped in on top of her feelings in a way that another person might not have. In a sense, she was arrogant with herself. In psychology, what Kathie did is called 'distancing'; she talked to herself as if she was another person, something we can and should tell our children to do from time to time. I'll have more to say about this, and other psychological hacks, in Part 3.

Your children are unlikely to have developed that sort of ability simply because they're children. It's mostly a very adult thing to be able to do. Nonetheless, you will have seen preschool children doing this. Sometimes they even invent imaginary friends whom they talk with. Later on, we will talk about the importance of learning to 'think twice' when faced with an adverse event. We need to teach our children that their first thoughts and feelings may not be accurate or proportional — particularly if they are associated with a bodily overreaction. If they are building up a number of distorted ways of seeing events, situations or occasions where they are becoming frightened in normal situations, they may need a spring clean to help them get rid of some of those bugs and imperfections that create biases in their thinking. That's where you come in, and where you can use your worldly powers to guide, facilitate and, indeed, instruct their thinking. As we have seen, this is not a mere matter of reassuring them: it is a matter of being their coach and psychological enabler.

Different courses for different horses

There are, in fact, more pathways that go up *from* the amygdala towards the cortex, meaning that our fear responses can overpower our rational responses. Can you see the problem with this? It means that we experience more fear than we'd like to and, at times, we will be trying to 'tamp down' our fear by using our mind, which can represent a real challenge. What a nuisance!

If you know how each pathway operates, you can help your child respond to an event in more adaptive ways. Unlike the cortex, the amygdala is not 'rational'; it's not good at thinking! For children, the amygdala's centre of gravity is in their bodies and not in their minds. Merely telling a child to *think* differently during an amygdala-fear event won't work. Similarly, telling a frightened child to just calm down or reassuring them won't necessarily work either.

People's well-intentioned logical responses to calm a child — like reassuring them — might not be the best solution to help a child who is experiencing fear. Rather, the therapy for fear-based anxiety involves a child learning ways to return to calm, using exercises that will calm their *body* down. We will learn about these body-reset techniques in Part 3.

For the moment, it is worth knowing that there are two places in a child's mind where they experience anxiety — and each needs to be soothed by distinct strategies.

In the next chapter we'll take a closer look at risks. We'll look at 'real' versus 'imagined' risks for children. My opinion on parents' perception of risk is that we've become more hesitant to let our children experience risk compared to when my kids were little. This can be a problem as far as children's mental health is concerned. It's not uncommon for us to react in favour of being safe if something is ambiguous. Some people would say we are making things too safe for children and that they can't do risky things any more. Doing risky things is important for a child so that they can learn from taking risks.

Did you know that salmon raised in fish farms are likely to die more quickly if they are subsequently put back in a river, compared with their river-raised cousins? Salmon raised on fish farms grow up 'predator naive'. That is, when they're overprotected in an environment that's too safe, they don't know how to operate in the natural environment. Had they grown up in the natural environment, they would have learnt three things: to stay away from the riverbank where bears would try to scoop them out of the water, to keep away from cod so they wouldn't be eaten, and to shoal, which is the fish version of 'safety in numbers'. In learning these three things they would survive longer and not be eaten![3]

Summary

» Stressors evoke an emotional response in any person. It's just that some people respond differently to the same stressors.

» Our assessment of an event or situation can be accurate or inaccurate. If cognitive distortions go unchecked, they can fuel anxiety.

» Knowing from where anxiety emanates can help us use the right techniques to treat that form of anxiety.

5.

What risk can we allow?

As we have seen, a central element in how we respond to a child who is experiencing anxiety is *how we compose ourselves* in important moments. If we see something as risky, we can prematurely jump in to stop something 'bad' from happening. The actual event may not be objectively 'bad' or risky — but we can find ourselves jumping in to protect our child because we might feel mean or negligent if we didn't. I get it; we want to protect our children from danger. But the problem is that we have become so cautious about some situations — and not others — that people are getting confused about what they will and won't let their children do.

There's no doubt that the number of activities we *perceive* as risky for our children has increased. When my children (now in their late 20s and early 30s) were in preschool, they could climb trees and play rough-and-tumble games. My wife and I allowed them to go bike riding in the neighbourhood, and to go to the skatepark and walk by themselves to the corner shop, from as young as seven or eight years old. From what I am hearing now, though, this type of behaviour is becoming increasingly suspect. In one Australian state that I know of, children can't legally walk to school alone under the age of 12 just in case something might happen to them.

My, how things have changed. My own mother and father had a very different approach. After school my father didn't worry himself about where my brothers or I were, as long as we were home before the streetlights came on. My mother had no idea where I was or what I was up to. Did this make either of them negligent? I don't think so. Was it safer back then than now? Again, I don't think so.

But what if all this recent worrying (by us) is negatively affecting our children's wellbeing? Because more people are perceiving greater risk than used to be the case, they are not letting their children do more adventurous or risky things. There is a cost for our children — and us — in this approach. It's important to know that some of our thinking about 'risk' is contextual. That is, we often won't allow for risky behaviour if we believe that the behaviour is frowned upon by our friends or by the wider community. In the space of one generation we may have become so hyper-aware of being judged that we have become risk averse! We might, in fact, be making our children nervous about things they don't need to be nervous about. I am not the only person seeing things this way.

In their book *The Coddling of the American Mind*, Jonathan Haidt and Greg Lukianoff say that a culture of 'safetyism' is making children more anxious. They say a culture of over-protectiveness is not only occurring on an individual level, but is now being put into law.

> 66 A culture that allows the concept of 'safety' to creep so far that it equates emotional discomfort with physical danger is a culture that encourages people to systematically protect one another from the very experiences embedded in daily life that they need, to become strong and healthy.[1]

In psychology, there is a concept called availability bias, which shows that when danger is available to view (for example, being all over the front page of the newspapers, such as when a child goes missing), we think it is more likely to happen to us — even if it is statistically unlikely. Availability bias is a mental shortcut we use to judge how likely it is something is going to happen based on how easily we can recall instances of it happening. Think top-of-mind images from the TV or the 'dagger' glances from other people in the supermarket if your child acts out of the ordinary. What do we do in these circumstances? Well, most people jump in to protect their child or stop the behaviour that's eliciting any of the 'dagger' looks from others. It's as if, if you're not super-careful all the time you run the risk of being accused of being irresponsible. Child protection agencies and media reports tell parents that they must care for their children in particular ways, lest they be seen as neglectful. All these phenomena — while well meaning — create the circumstances for anxious parenting.

So where does this leave us? Do we simply let our children roam free and do more risky things? Will we be judged as negligent if we allow our children to experience risk by not intervening? Will we be held accountable for not acting to protect children when others think we should have?

Unless children gain real-life experience at solving real-life problems they are not likely to develop emotional resilience. Remember what Taleb said? Some things get better and stronger when put to the test.

For yourself, once you have worked out that your child's tree-climbing or solo visit to the shops represents a small risk, you will have to develop 'nonchalance'.

It's important to have a plan for what you will and won't jump in on to protect them or get upset on their behalf about. The action of writing this down will stop you acting inadvertently. Sorting out what is too-risky versus what's not-too-risky will help you to control your own reactions. That's what we're going to do now. It's one of the most important jobs you'll do in this book, so let's take the time to work out how to do it properly.

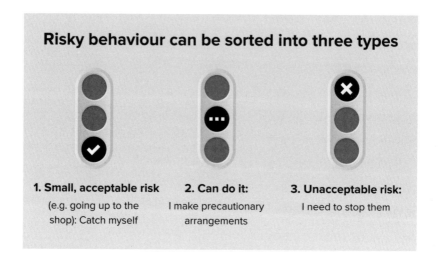

Risky behaviour can be sorted into three types

1. Small, acceptable risk:
(e.g. going up to the shop): Catch myself

2. Can do it:
I make precautionary arrangements

3. Unacceptable risk:
I need to stop them

How to sort risk

To sort risks, follow the steps below.

1. Observe your child's behaviour and activities over a week or so. Try to observe at least six behaviours or activities.

2. Now discuss your child's behaviours and activities with any significant adults in your household. What do you agree are the levels of risk for each of these? The three categories for behaviours and activities/events are: small acceptable risks, about which you will do nothing (e.g. using a knife in the kitchen); not too risky, for which you will make some precautionary arrangements (e.g. a sleepover at a friend's house); and unacceptable risks, for which the answer is 'no' (e.g. not letting your eleven-year-old daughter go to an unsupervised teenage party).

3. Now look at the table below. Sort the six behaviours and activities into the three columns, reflecting on what you discussed in the previous step.

Small, acceptable risk — I ignore these	Not too risky — I make pre-cautionary arrangements	Unacceptable risks — the answer is 'no'

You may wish to see how your responses compare with other parents' responses. Let's look at how some parents I have trained have completed each of the columns. But first, let me say if you found this exercise hard to do, you're not alone! This sorting task can be really difficult, because most parents err on the side of risk aversion. It's very difficult to know what kinds of risks we 'can allow' or 'not allow'.

Of course, what you will and won't let your child do will also depend on their age. You wouldn't let your four-year-old cross a road to go to the shop by themselves, but you might let your eight-year-old do that. And you would not involve a child in taking sides in an argument between you and your partner. You'd hopefully try to work out those types of problems in private, away from young ears.

The key point in doing the sorting exercise is that children need to take some risks — and it's good for them to do so. But clearly, there are some things you'll need to protect them from. With small risks, you'll need to practise your nonchalance! With larger risks, you'll need to say 'no'. Keep in mind, too, that what you consider acceptable will change as your child grows, so you will need to periodically reassess and amend your expectations around risk.

By writing down these activities, you're actively considering the risks and you'll be more conscious of the choices you make. This process will help you become more automatic about what you'll ignore and what you'll take precautions about. Once you can identify something as only slightly risky, you can manage your own impulses to step in. Your self-talk here is going to be important so that you don't let your feelings get in the way. I know that life can become busy but there will be times when you'll have to have a good talk to yourself. You'll need to remind yourself, 'I don't need to jump in on this occasion; she'll work it out if I give her the space.'

It is one thing to have a list of situations for which you say to yourself you're going to allow this or that to happen or ignore certain things; it is quite another thing to stop yourself from jumping in to protect your child.

My half tongue-in-cheek message to you earlier in this chapter about developing your nonchalance is important. On one hand, you may, in theory, allow certain behaviour to take place. However, if your facial expressions tell your child you are still worried about them doing certain things, it's likely this will play a significant role in whether or not your child will 'have a go'. After all, actions speak louder than words.

The Cooper family's risk-sorting task

Here are some typical risks Jane and Andrew found when doing their sorting task:

Small, acceptable risk (ignore these):

- Tom can climb a tree by himself.
- Tom can play rugby.

- Tom can use a knife unaided in the kitchen.
- Both Tom and Emma can go and borrow something from the neighbours (e.g. rice or sugar).
- Both can go to the shop to make a purchase.
- Both can talk with strangers (especially when one of us is there).
- Both can wait at the front of the shop reading their book while one of us is finishing the shopping.
- We will allow both to struggle (emotionally) with a dilemma that it is within their grasp to wrestle with.
- Both can wait in the car while one of us pays for petrol.

Not too risky (make precautionary arrangements):

- Sleepover at a friend's house (but we will call the friend's parents first).
- Ride their bikes to school (we've trained them and ridden with them a few times already).
- Go with their mates on a bike ride around the block (we know this will be okay because we know our neighbourhood).

- Tom can go to the skatepark with his mates by himself (there are lots of other children down at the park on weekends).

Unacceptable risk (no):

- Sleepover at a house when there are no parents at home.
- Allowing Emma to go to a teenage party where we know they'll be drinking.
- Allowing Emma or Tom to use social apps (like Instagram) before they are thirteen and which we know are not good for their mental health.
- Any activity that involves breaking the law.
- Staying up past 8 p.m. to play digital games on a regular school night.

Postscript on sorting behaviour

There's a growing movement to allow children to experience more risk. On this note, I recommend you have a look at Lenore Skenazy's website www.letgrow.org. It contains lots of research about real versus imagined risk for children.

In Part 3, I will show you a selection of 'modest' strategies that you can use to help your children manage anxiety. But before we get 'on the tools', there's one more piece of the puzzle I'd like to spend some time on — how family patterns become established and, just as importantly, how to *change* patterns in a family.

Summary

» Realize that it is important for your child to face some risky situations — including friendship problems — without you jumping in to fix things.

» Realize that if your child is to become more resilient, they need to not just tolerate some pain but also to be given the processes to enable them to handle adversity.

» Sort behaviour into three types: small, acceptable risks (where you will do nothing), not-too-risky (where you take reasonable precautions), and unacceptable risks (where you say 'no').

PART 2

Modifying anxiety over time

The next two chapters examine the reasons why patterns become entrenched in families. Here we'll focus on what parents can be tempted to do and what results from their behaviour, and we begin to unpack what happens for your child when *you* begin to change your behaviour. At times, you won't be able to change your child's behaviour — but you will be able to change your own.

6.

Patterns in families and how to change them

Systems operate all around us. We have transport, weather, banking and health systems. There are circulatory systems in our bodies. All these systems have one thing in common: they have parts that work together, usually with predictable things happening one after the other. For example, there is a predictable pattern in a transport system. At certain times of the day more trains will run. There will be fewer trains running at other times, such as late at night. If a train breaks down in one part of the system, it will delay other trains.

Let me give you my own definition of a system: 'A system is a collection of parts that operate together in a sequenced way.' One of the systems I talk about with parents is a car engine. A car engine is made up of various parts: spark plugs, fuel, battery, leads and so on. Take the battery out and the engine won't work. Drain the fuel out and the engine won't work. Remove the spark plugs and the engine won't work. But if you take one spark plug out, what will happen? Well, the engine will function differently. It will still work but it will chug along very roughly! Each of the different parts of the engine relies on the other parts to make the engine work as a system. If you tinker with one part of a car engine it will affect the other parts. That's the way systems work; all the parts of the system are interdependent.

From a systems perspective, we can observe certain patterns occurring in a family. If something has happened 100 times, we can assume it will occur 101 times. Psychologists who work with families have shown that once patterns get established in families, they tend to stay the same for long periods until something or somebody makes them operate differently. For example, family systems change when children turn into teenagers. Teenagers want more privacy; they'll also want to spend more time with their mates and less time with their parents.

As a child grows older, their experience is made up of little incidents and episodes of anxiety, which can become patterned. A pattern can form when a child develops a fear of something like fire (e.g. they become fixated on anything to do with fire) and then they avoid other feared situations (e.g. going in lifts or being afraid of heights). When a group of fixations becomes pronounced, the child might stop doing anything that could result in them feeling fear or uncertainty. Hopefully, your child won't reach anything resembling a big problem with anxiety, and you wouldn't want them to. But if you can 'see' the early signs of anxious behaviour in a child — and if you can get 'in there' to turn things around — you can help them develop more courage and bravery.

Let's look at how a pattern has been established in the Cooper family.

- Not for the first time, Tom has a bad day at school — he had an argument with a friend.
- The next day, Tom says he doesn't want to go to school.
- At first, Jane says, 'No, you're going to go to school!'
- Tom catastrophizes and creates a scene.
- Jane relinquishes and lets Tom stay home.
- Tom plays on his device all day.

In pictorial form, this is how the above pattern looks:

Patterns follow a sequence

Tom has a bad day at school

Tom says he doesn't want to go

Tom plays on device all day

Jane says, 'You have to go.'

Jane concedes & relinquishes

Tom catastrophises & creates a scene

Problem solved...until next time!

While knowing it would be better for all concerned if Tom went to school, Jane gives in to Tom's wishes because to insist seems either too harsh or that it would cause too much drama.

In this case, being too harsh or creating too much drama is not the main problem. We know *why* these types of patterns occur. In the short-term, there are wins for both. Things are immediately more pleasant for both parties: Tom has avoided going to school and, by giving in, Jane has stopped the drama. But, long-term, a pattern is maintained. In this case, short-term rewards are paid for by longer-term unpleasant consequences. Jane has increased the likelihood that Tom will behave like this in the future. And Jane will tend to give in next time because she would feel *mean* if she doesn't.

Children have two systems for managing anxiety. They have an independent system, where they can learn to 'get back to calm' under their own steam. And they have an attachment system, where they can use a parent to help them get back to calm. The thing is that anxious children can try to involve parents in seeking to *avoid* a problem they do not want to face.

'Family accommodation' of childhood anxiety is the term used to describe the *changes* parents make to their behaviour (and their family's living patterns) due to a child's anxious behaviour.

Parents can be overinfluenced to change their family routines (e.g. to stop going out) or they can end up joining in with their children's anxious behaviour (e.g. obsessively washing hands). Eli Lebowitz explains how more and more parents (and an increasing number of teachers, for that matter) are accommodating children's anxiety rather than helping a child to engage with life's normal stresses.[1] That is, when children put up even an ounce of resistance to engaging with life's normal challenges, an increasing number of parents are tending to give in to the child's reluctance where once they would not have. And, once we start doing that many times over many years, two things occur: children learn that by behaving anxiously they can *avoid* events, occasions or situations, and parents inadvertently contribute to their child developing cognitive distortions. The child learns to exaggerate and misinterpret otherwise-neutral cues as danger signals. When parents accommodate, 'they unconsciously obscure a child's ability to correctly label anxious thoughts as unrealistic or exaggerated'.[2] Wow, huh?

In the example of the Coopers above, Tom's avoiding behaviour is negatively reinforced. Instead of rummaging in a kit bag of different ways in which he can (independently) face the challenge of going to school, his mother instead rescues him by once again aiding him to avoid something that is within his ability to face. At a subliminal level, he makes a proverbial mountain out of a molehill. The more he does that across his childhood, the more he is reinforced to behave anxiously.

So that you don't think cognitive distortions are all down to parents, I'd like to alert you to the fact that, in a culture of 'safetyism', it's not just parents who are doing the accommodating and aiding and abetting anxiety in children; it's also some school systems and some teachers who are contributing to this problem. Over the past five years, I've heard many teachers complain about the number of times children are being excused for opting out or not attending school by GPs and mental and allied health professionals. This places teachers and educators in a difficult position. They don't feel that they can or should question the advice given by mental health professionals. Teachers tell me that some registered mental health professionals are supplying parents with 'stay-at-home' letters or calling on schools not to 'stress' a child because of their anxiety. These pieces of advice are supplied to the school in the expectation that the school won't place extraordinary demands on a child and to help them avoid what could be objectively considered moderate-level challenges.

In some instances, these opt-out alternatives are provided without a treatment plan from the mental health professional to help the child return to the classroom. Teachers also tend to give in to this advice because they fear the blowback they will get from parents if they don't. However, it is also the case that far more children are being allowed to absent themselves for weaker reasons than ever before.

I can see why this is happening: mental health professionals want to be compassionate and perhaps give a child time to regroup. However, if the child has mild anxiety they shouldn't be acting contrary to the best clinical advice for treating mild anxiety in children, which is *not* to accommodate anxiety. Rather, the best clinical advice is to devise treatment plans to help a child overcome a mental health impairment. And these steps to help children overcome their anxious habits should be communicated to parents, teachers and school systems so that everybody is pulling in the same direction.

Children need those around them to not just support them to manage their anxious feelings, but also to help them actively engage with adversity. According to Lebowitz, there is now ample research to show that 'coping with moderate levels of anxiety in the context of healthy and supportive adult relationships actually increases a child's coping skills and promotes resilience'.[3]

When the significant adults in a child's life *identify* anxious behaviour, they need to 'stop the bus' and intervene when the child's anxiety is getting the better of them. This is not just about helping a child feel better in the moment (though that should be a long-term outcome). Rather, it involves adults helping a child to learn the skills to solve emotional problems and, when needed, to use arousal reduction skills to reduce their physical symptoms.

Unfortunately, the longer a child's anxiety is accommodated — and the more they are helped to avoid life's normal challenges — the worse their anxiety tends to become. The more everyone around an anxious child backs off (often for fear of pushing and making things worse), the more likely it is that a child's mental health will deteriorate. For parents, this can be a hard pattern to reverse out of. I've seen many parents face significant challenges — including child aggression — when they try to change a pattern of accommodation. To a child who has been accommodated for years, their parents behaving differently can appear like mutiny.

In these instances, the child has become used to a pattern of behaviour where the parent normally gives in.

What children learn from parents' reactions

Following is a list of what a child *learns* from a parent's reaction. For example, Emma has 'learnt' that if she gets herself in a 'state', her parents will sometimes give in to her franticness. She has also learnt that if she invites her mother to do her work for her, her mother will oblige. Tom has learnt that he gets attention from his mother by repeatedly asking his mother for reassurance. He has also learnt that he only has to protest in the slightest possible manner to get to stay home from school. Emma has learnt that by protesting going out to restaurants she can 'make' her parents change their minds.

Signs of anxious behaviour	What the child says or does	What parents might normally do
Emma 'feels' distressed in her body and becomes fretful, frantic or volatile.	'I can't do that! No, no I can't just "feel" this way.' (She reels from the event/situation.)	Jane placates, distracts or gives in to Emma. Becomes exasperated.
Tom pesters his mother to ensure she's going to 'be there'.	Tom keeps asking, 'Are you sure you'll be there?'	Jane keeps reassuring Tom, saying, 'Yes, I'll be there.'
Emma invites Jane to do her school project.	Emma says, 'Can you do it for me?' (When Jane doesn't, Emma gets more upset.)	Jane might normally jump in to fix things. She doesn't want to risk a drama and ends up doing the task for Emma.
Tom 'avoids' friendship problems by not going to school.	Tom 'locks down' quickly on a 'no'. He forms a habit of catastrophizing.	Andrew helps Tom avoid a challenging situation by letting him stay home.
Emma doesn't want to go to places or do normal family things. Her bandwidth of 'normal' narrows.	Emma avoids participating in normal tasks. She wants her parents to agree not to do certain things.	Jane and Andrew 'accommodate' by changing a family routine e.g. not eating out at restaurants.

What the child learns from the parents' reaction	Teach the child a coping micro-skill instead
Emma learns that losing control of her body (hyperventilating) is acceptable.	
Tom learns that his distress will be smoothed over by someone else's reassurance.	
Emma learns that 'small' problems cannot be managed by herself.	
Tom learns that challenging tasks are to be avoided.	
Emma learns that her emotional distress is stronger than she is able to control.	

Changing patterns

Even if your child is temperamentally anxious, they can learn new ways of doing things to manage their anxiety. Despite an anxious temperament, your child will need to know how to get on in the world. It's the same for children who have special needs, such as those with a diagnosis of ADHD (Attention Deficit Hyperactivity Disorder) or those who are on the autism spectrum. I tell parents this: 'Even though he is *not* neuro-typical, he will need to learn how to control his impulsiveness at school. It'll be a bit harder for him, but he can learn some self-control strategies. I can show you some.'

For the most part, the things we fear — or the anxiety we experience in life — don't necessarily go away. As we grow older, we frame things differently compared to children simply because we gain more perspective.

As far as anxiety is concerned, it's more likely that we will always become alarmed in certain situations and we're likely to still panic in others. What can and does change is our ability to *manage* fears or anxious thoughts. This is a good way of thinking about anxiety. It de-pathologizes it. And it makes it everyone's business. It means that if we can all learn strategies to manage our own natural reactions to stresses, we can transfer those same skills to help our children. Unless someone shows a child how to manage their fears and anxious thoughts, they won't necessarily learn them by osmosis. Because we know a lot more about *how* anxiety can be controlled these days, we can do more than our parents did.

I compare learning to control anxiety as being akin to learning wrestling-holds to overpower an opponent. When I was a teenager in the 1970s (I know that's going back a while) I, like many boys my age, would watch World Championship Wrestling on the TV. We watched the likes of Mario Milano, Skull Murphy and Killer Kowalski. The commentators referred to these wrestlers' holds with names like 'the claw', the 'half-nelson', and the 'headlock'. Where am I going with this? Well, anxiety is something like that for children. They can get better at wrestling with their anxious feelings or thoughts, and they can even learn ways to wrestle with their amygdala!

The key message for children is that anxiety is surmountable — and under their control. As we learnt in the last chapter, quite a few anxious patterns get set up in even well-meaning and loving families. Every parent loves their children, and every parent does not want their children to suffer unnecessarily. Where a pattern has been established in a family for a long time, it can feel like groundhog day and mightily inconvenient if a child's anxiety results in changes that interfere with a family's normal functioning. For example, at the moment the Coopers can't or won't go out because of Emma's anxiety.

Change processes — and how they work

We've all seen situations of behaviour change being used by governments or companies to either positively affect public health outcomes or to make a company's processes more efficient. My own story of change involves being trained by a company to follow a new process it wanted its customers to use. It involved me learning how to implement a new ticketing system at my local airport in the early 2000s. At the time, my preferred airline was attempting to change the behaviour of tens of thousands of passengers by introducing a new self-check-in process. So they were proactive in approaching people. Every time I entered the terminal, on my way to the customer service line, a member of the airline's ground crew approached me, saying, 'Hello sir, can I show you how to use our new self-check-in facility?' The crew member correspondingly pointed at the machine. 'Do you have a booking number?'

Because I was used to being checked in at the service counter, I resisted the staff member's efforts to bring me into the 21st century! Grimacing slightly, I would ask, 'Is there someone I can be served by instead?' Each time I subsequently went to the airport, something similar happened: 'Sir, can I help you? Can I show you how to use the self-check-in kiosk?'

This new way of doing things was unfamiliar to me and I wasn't sure if I could do what was required. The first few times I was asked to join in I was not motivated to overcome my mental block at being asked to do so. In the back of my mind, I was saying to myself, 'Here is a company trying to get me to do part of their work.' I was also 'thinking' those people (behind the counter) are going to lose their jobs. But a third part of my resistance, if I am to be truthful, was that I was not confident about using the touchscreen on the device. You would have observed me to be reluctant, disengaged and apathetic. My facial expressions would have been blank and my body posture closed. All the outward signs would have reflected a lack of enthusiasm for the job at hand. On later occasions, though, if I had more time, the ground crew were more easily able to engage me. 'I'm not in a rush,' I'd think, 'so, why not?' Each time the staff member's approach was the same, and each time I agreed to be engaged I learnt more about what was going on. The airline was getting me used to what it wanted me to do. The staff reassured and coached me. Slowly but surely, I was being cajoled and encouraged to change over to the new system.

Eventually, the staff trained me so well that when other people from my office accompanied me to training workshops, I would sometimes try to train them to use the self-check-in kiosks: 'Do you know how to do this? I do! Come over here and I'll help you!' The airline's goal was to make the use of its self-check-in system the 'normal' way of doing things, changing the behaviour of tens of thousands of passengers in the process. The airline's management knew this was going to take time and effort. It knew that not everyone would welcome this and it would have to persevere in training its staff to deal with resistant customers like me. The airline knew that it didn't have to achieve everything at once. It couldn't.

Let's talk about me. If you were a fly on the wall, what do you think you would have noticed? I was hesitant and resistant to change. While I wasn't rude to anyone, my body language would have conveyed that I was a reluctant participant in what they were trying to do. Clearly, the airline's staff would encounter a wide range of customers — young people, elderly people, people experienced in using touchscreens and some people with no experience. Some customers no doubt would have had even stronger views than I did about doing a corporation's work for them. Others, like me, just preferred being served by real people.

Now, let's talk about the airline. What did they do well? Well, you would have observed that they were consistent. In fact, each time I went to the airport it was the same message every time. They were persistent. They didn't just try once; their effort wasn't just a once-off. They persevered. On separate occasions, there may have been different people approaching me, and they might have expressed what they were trying to achieve in slightly different ways, but their message was similar. This is a good example of 'same skeleton, different coat'!

The best change efforts I have seen tend to involve several factors: good initial training of staff about the objective of the change initiative, training simulations including role plays, identification of the likely blocks in people's willingness to cooperate (and how to overcome them), and making the steps in the process easy to do. When staff are being trained to implement a strategy like this, they are shown what their script is and how to implement the strategy. Each step in the change process is important in and of itself and, in combination, the steps will have more effect than if you did just one of the steps on its own.

Take the Australian government's attempt to reduce the road toll over the past 40 years, for example. (Apparently, Australia is world famous for this change project.) In the 1980s the road toll was unacceptably high, with 43.5 deaths per 100,000 vehicles on the road. The cost in terms of human suffering alone was enormous and simply terrible for those families involved. The state road safety people knew what would make the biggest difference in lowering the road toll — and they kept going on about those same things as many times as they could. They focused on high impact techniques or activities, year after year and decade after decade, and eventually they lowered the road toll to 3.9 deaths per 100,000 vehicles on the road.

By changing the laws for speeding and drink driving, by fixing roads and by making cars safer, and through public education campaigns, they decreased the road toll. With limited resources (taxpayer dollars), the people initiating the changes knew they had to invest in high-efficacy initiatives rather than assuming that all initiatives were equally helpful. Anyway, you get my drift. If you want to impact your child's anxiousness, you'd do well to attack the problem from different angles. When it comes to changing a pattern within your family, I want you to remember this: children often think in the moment, but you need to think in terms of weeks and months. Just as the airline's ground crew had a long-term plan about how to change its customers' behaviour, and just as the road-toll project leaders came at the same problem through multiple pathways, so you, too, need to take a longer-term view of change. Knowing about how change occurs is important because if you know that it will take some time, you will persevere.

When it comes to changing a pattern in your family you will need to remember that your child will not necessarily welcome a new way of doing things. Just as the airline got some resistance from me, so, too, your children will resist a new way of doing things, simply because they are used to things occurring in a particular way. If you're going to change your child's anxious behaviour it is likely that your child will struggle a bit — at least in the beginning.

The one person you have control over is yourself. Remember I said to you that the approach in *The Anxiety Coach* involves you doing *less* of some things and *more* of others? You will need to behave towards your children like the airline staff behaved towards me — by being persistent, calm and helpful but not accommodating. Even if it takes time to see improvements, you shouldn't be discouraged or tempted to revert to old habits such as over-reassuring or solving problems for them. If you're consistent, you will see positive changes happening. As it turns out, there are only a few changes that you will need to be consistent about. These modest changes, over time, will work.

A couple of years back, the Canadian psychologist Jordan Peterson wrote the book *12 Rules for Life*. In his chapter on child-rearing, he said that many parents he'd seen were very hands off. They tried not to influence their children in any way, leaving them in an undifferentiated state: 'Children are damaged when those charged with their care, afraid of any conflict or upset, no longer dare to correct them and leave them without guidance.'[4] So, according to Peterson, by not acting and by not 'attending incisively' at various junctures in a child's behaviour, many parents are leaving their children to fend for themselves. Peterson reckoned this was not good.

I agree with his views about there being a lack of incisive attention being used by parents. Here are a few ways of looking at this problem.

First, when it comes to anxiety, some of us believe it is not our place or our role to correct our children's faulty thinking. We don't see ourselves as our children's trainers in this way. So, without knowing what else to do, we find ourselves paralyzed. Then we end up giving in to our children's wishes to avoid an anxiety-provoking situation, simply because it's easier. If you don't see one of your roles as being your child's coach (see Chapter 3) you simply won't do it.

Second, some of us see that challenging children about their anxious talking or anxious behaviour feels mean. It is a very difficult thing to do to stand by and watch a child go through a difficult emotion without wanting to step in to take pain away from them. We might want to do something, anything, to relieve their pain.

Third, many parents lack an alternative plan for managing a child's anxiety. And without a well-learned process, it's really hard not to be overcome by our own feelings that we're somehow being mean. I've seen this enough to think it's true. Many parents won't act to help a child wrestle with their feelings because they don't have a go-to replacement process or they are just too worried about a child being 'uncomfortable'. They let their own feelings (of not wanting to upset their child) get in the road of helping their child build their resilience skills.

I am not being a proponent of 'tough love' parenting here. That's not what I am saying. However, I *am* saying children need to be challenged to become better problem-solvers and to learn how to question their initial feelings so that they can learn to modify their emotional reactions. All these skills are within the grasp of the average child to learn but they require a parent to be proactive.

If you can freeze-frame a situation when your child is anxious and give them your attention, you can really help them to manage their anxiety, not just for now, but into the future. If you repeat this process, you can facilitate their ability to cope with adversity.

The Coopers recognized that they could not go on with their children the way things were going. While Emma was a lovely girl in herself, they also saw how she could be her own worst enemy. They loved her bubbly, effervescent nature. However, they also noticed she tended to create problems for herself (and her parents) by becoming heightened and frantic, and by wanting things to be just right. They wanted her to take more risks and to 'have a go' at things, even if these were not in her comfort zone. Rather than habitually locking down on a hard 'no' if things looked challenging, they wanted her to 'think again' and reconsider. They also wanted Emma to develop her psychological core strength so that she did not fall apart or appear as fragile as she had been.

Changes in anyone's behaviour rarely go smoothly. It's not usually a straightforward thing. The Coopers needed to know that the road ahead might not be smooth to begin with. Thousands of experiments by behavioural scientists say the same thing: people (including children) don't like change, but they will generally adapt with time and perseverance from the 'change agent'. In this case, that's you. And that has to be worth the initial resistance, doesn't it?

In the Cooper household, Emma's behaviour had been accommodated for many years. Tom also had been told again and again (reassured) that he would be picked up from after-school activities. As a result, Jane and Andrew knew that it would be tricky to reverse out of a pattern they had unwittingly established. They knew they would have to play the short game and the long game. The short game would involve them responding to Emma and Tom's anxiety by using opportunities presented to them to help their children to reframe how they reacted to different events. The long game, they knew, involved them effectively modifying previously held ways in which they responded to Emma and Tom.

In the coming chapters, I will start laying out the tools for change. These are the 'modest' tools I referred to earlier. They are truly easy to learn and use. If you know which tool to use, and when to use it, it will help.

Summary

» When behaviour patterns get established, they become a bit more predictable. If they have happened 100 times, they are likely to happen 101 times.

» Parents can inadvertently contribute to a pattern of anxiety — through a process called accommodation — by either changing their own behaviour (e.g. not going out) or by *joining in* with a child's behaviour (such as overwashing hands).

» Change takes time. Change works better when you come at what you're trying to change from different angles.

7.

A quick overview and the elements of good design

Let's catch up on where we've been and take a sneak peek at where we are going to in coming chapters.

In Part 1 of the book, we looked at some important knowledge points: the importance of developing an internal locus of control and its benefits for children, the way in which resilience can be 'constructed', and how we can overcome our doubts. We saw that the role of the coach is to teach micro-skills. We identified that anxiety comes in two forms: anxious thoughts and images, and fear. The origin-points for these different types of anxiety are important to know if we are to support a child to outwit their anxiety. We learnt that most anxious behavior in children is learnt over time — and it can become a pattern. So the good news is that if a pattern is learnt, it can be changed. What we saw in the previous chapter is that change can take time — and it can involve some disruption while you attempt to create a new pattern.

Up to this point, our intervention design has largely been of a 'what you would do less of' type. So by reassuring less, by not allowing your child to avoid too much and by reducing accommodation, you can reduce anxiety and develop your child's resilience over months and years. I am not being heartless here. Of course, there will be times when your child will need your support and even your reassurance. But I'm asking you to put your 'objective' hat on if you see your child behaving anxiously. Being objective means that you will see your child's behaviour for what it is — and you'll be aiming to help them manage their anxiety and not be swayed to acquiesce or help them avoid something difficult.

Hopefully, your reassurance will be *less* of the type that implies 'Here, I will fix it for you' and *more* of the type that indicates 'I think you've got this'. This 'less of' orientation is something that is under *your* control, and it will involve you taking more control of *your own behaviour* so that it doesn't have an effect on your child's anxious behaviour. Eli Lebowtiz's big finding about child anxiety is that the more the child is prompted to rely on their own resources, the less anxious and more resourceful they will become.

From here on in, until the end of the book, I'm going to show you some of the 'more of' elements of what you can do to reduce your child's anxious behaviour. This will involve you becoming better at objectifying when your child is behaving anxiously and then working out what you will do to support and challenge them to behave less anxiously. By assuming an objective pose and setting your own feelings to the side, your job is to become your child's coach. Again, what does the coach do? *He or she teaches the micro-skill in the micro-moment.*

You can provide your child with the scaffolds they'll need to develop mental blueprints to manage adversity. These blueprints might be light blue to begin with. But with your help and confidence in your child's ability to cope, they will get more defined over time.

Two modes for helping your child

There are two main ways to consider your role as an initiator in improving your child's ability to manage anxiety: the first is when you will 'strike when the iron is hot' and the other is when you will 'strike when the iron is cold'.[1]

Striking while the iron is *hot* is knowing what script to follow in 'serve and return' conversations so that you don't fall into the trap of accommodating but you do know how to respond. Your child 'serves' you an anxious thought or behaviour, now what do you do? You need to respond. As we saw in the chart on p. 87, Andrew and Jane's responses might be easy in the short term. However, the more their responses inadvertently help their children to avoid using an internal locus of control approach, the more their children's external locus of control settings will become a pattern.

Instead, by asking a child to catch their thoughts and to reconsider them, you can help them develop more adaptive narrative structures. You can help them to develop more constructive ways of describing events to themselves. But wait, there's more! You can also help them get into the new habit of thinking again — of not taking things at face value — and developing the habit of reworking an event from a scientific viewpoint. The acronym SALON, which I first introduced to you on p. 8, is our main tool for holding this type of conversation.

When your child plays an anxious curveball 'at' you, you might be tempted to reassure, placate or distract them. While this might be the *natural* thing to do, it's not necessarily the *best* thing to do — at least not on its own. In fact, as a school principal once told me, if you immediately shift a child away from working through their anxiousness too quickly, you're 'stealing the moment' from them. The child won't have the opportunity to wrestle with their problem. These exchanges need not be long ones. I'm not talking about 'therapy' here. Even in the briefest encounters an adult can support a child to think in scientific ways, so they learn how to be accurate, proportional and realistic (not fatuous, disproportionate and unrealistic). These can be brief encounters, but they need to be regular and consistent ones.

Remember what the airline staff did with me? They were able to get me to change my behaviour in two-minute encounters.

So, too, with your children; you will need to support them across several conversations to embed in them better ways for them to wrestle with their anxious thoughts and feelings. We're going to be covering one of these encounters with a worked example from the Cooper family in Part 3.

Striking while the iron is *cold* is teaching them how to use strategies long known by psychologists to help a child regulate ruminating or heightened bodily reactions. The aim here is to teach your child how to cope with a *future* event. These are pre-taught — meaning that you are teaching them this skill for when a future episode of anxiety occurs. These types of interventions include arousal reduction techniques and interrupting techniques to stop mental cycling. We're also going to be covering these in Part 3.

Whether you're using a strike when the iron is hot mode or teaching your child when the iron is cold, you'll need to remember, they are both *processes*. If you learn these processes, you will remember them when you need to use them.

Of course, whether you respond to a child's anxiety might simply depend on a judgment call you'll make at the time. It might not be the best time, right there and then, to stop everything to attend to your child's anxiousness. You might need to have been somewhere five minutes ago and you don't want to run any later than you already are. Or you might have guests coming over. And then there are small anxieties you might not want to treat in the same way you treat bigger ones. Or you yourself are not in the right frame of mind to be the coach. What I am saying is that, just as with risky behaviour, you might let some anxious moments 'go through to the keeper' or slide at that particular time. You can pick and choose your moment to intervene. Over the medium term, though, you shouldn't let their anxious or distorted talking 'go' past you too many times.

The through-theme of our intervention is that you will have expectations of your child and your family:

» Your family will be a 'have a go' family — and everyone behaves accordingly.

» It's *your* job (not someone else's) to promote your child's independence and to 'prepare them for the road'.

» Your child will learn to think about things accurately and proportionately. No use of catastrophizing or emotional reasoning where it's not warranted.

The following strategies are the spine of our intervention. Each of these by themselves will make a difference to your child's anxiety (that's what the research evidence shows); in combination, they will be even more powerful.

» **Mind maintenance.** Help your child maintain good levels of brain-readiness through good sleep habits, through your management of technology at home, through looking 'at' them in the eye, and getting out in nature.

» **Skill them in ways to tame their fears**. Help children to face their fears by using graded exposure techniques.

» **Listen to them more.** Acknowledge, validate and support your child, without resorting to over-reassuring or giving in to their anxious behaviour.

» **Help them to think more accurately.** Help your child assess situations more proportionally using SALON.

PART 3

The Anxiety Coach tactics

The six chapters in this part of the book offer strategies for helping a child to develop advanced skills in overcoming fear and anxious thinking. Here we will focus on the modest skills any parent can use to help their child deal with stress and adversity. The highlight tactic in this part is SALON. By repeating parts of all the tactics, but especially SALON, your child will improve their internal locus of control skills.

8.

Mind maintenance

To support your child's ability to manage stress, you need to make sure that their mind is working properly. If your child's mind was a widget (a small but important mechanical part of a larger machine), you would want that widget to be operating efficiently.

In us all, our mind has a particular job of coordinating incoming information (from our senses: seeing, hearing, smelling, etc.) and it makes sense of situations, events or problems. This coordinating only happens optimally if the neural machinery is in good condition. In adults, assuming our mind is in good shape (it's well rested and in good mental health) it can usually sort out confusing or ambiguous problems and organize a proportional response to adverse events. There is a developmental aspect to a child's increasing ability to respond to a stressor, but there is also a learnt aspect to our mind's ability to organize a proportional response. So a child's response will get better (the older they become) and the more that those around them hold expectations that the child can work things out.

In experiments where researchers have divided children into anxious and non-anxious groups, even the non-anxious children tend to get more anxious than adults. Children's minds are still learning to cope with stress and they're not as good at it when compared with adults. This finding also infers that an adult needs to actively construct a child's environment so that their fledgling abilities can develop.

Look after their sleep habits

There is a copious amount of evidence for why getting good sleep is a necessary part of helping your child with their anxiety.[1] The ability of children's minds to respond to anxious thoughts or fears is even less effective if they don't sleep properly.[2] So for a child's mind to be operating at full tilt it needs to be well rested, and this — my dear parent — is where you come in! You'll need to set up rules for when your child goes to bed and when they get up. Getting this right will translate into them not just being better equipped to manage anxiety, it will help them to manage any behavioural meltdowns as well.

When parents come to see me about a child's anxiety, you might be surprised to know that one of my first ports of call is how much sleep their child is getting. Much of a child's anxiety is tied up with their quantity and quality of sleep. What psychologists notice is that a child's anxiety 'presentation' often has as much to do with a lack of timely, uninterrupted sleep as it does with anything else. The guidelines on sleep hygiene are pretty good these days. Here, you can see what sleep children of different ages should be getting. Get 'good sleep' right and your efforts will reduce your child's anxiety.

Sleep

HOW MUCH SLEEP DO WE NEED?

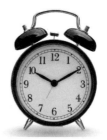

- **Babies under 1:** 14-18 hours throughout the day and night
- **Toddlers:** 12-14 hours per 24 hour period
- **Primary school:** 10-12 hours per day
- **High school:** 9-11 hours per day
- **Adults:** 7-9 hours per day

Sleepeducation.net.au/sleep%20facts.php

Children who don't sleep well can't as effectively do battle with their amygdala. As we saw in the chapter on anxiety basics, a child's amygdala can send fear messages up neural pathways. If children's minds aren't rested, they can't tamp down an 'up-regulating' limbic response. Matthew Walker, from Berkeley University, found that without proper sleep, the brain reverts to more primitive patterns of activity in that it can't put emotional experiences into context and produce a controlled, proportional response. Those last five words are important: *produce a controlled, proportional response.* The effect of a lack of sleep is that the limbic system tends to up-regulate — meaning that it pushes up the neuronal pathways from the 'old' brain. What then happens is that the child can't respond well.

Take some control over their access to the internet

When I run workshops on children's use of technology, I talk with parents about technology and its place in the home. I refer to the internet as an 'invited guest', not an assumed resident at your house — which ultimately means you may not have control over what happens 'out there' on the net, but you can control what happens in your home because it has big implications for protecting your child's mental wellbeing. There's also growing evidence that unbridled access to applications such as video games or social media platforms affects children's mental health.[3]

You have bought this book because your child is under thirteen years of age. This is the time when many children begin asking parents for their own personal device, typically a smartphone — which involves access to the worldwide web, social apps, and a treasure trove of great and also damaging features. I am not saying tweens shouldn't use these apps. That would be unrealistic. Screen-based media use is a hot topic when it comes to parenting. Over the past decade, I have been advised by my fellow mental health professionals, some of whom specialize in children's and young people's digital usage, that anyone giving advice to parents about children's digital usage needs to be encouraging children to become responsible users of technology. At face value, this seems reasonable advice.

The advice of my colleagues goes along the lines that we can't ban devices, so we have to teach them how to use their devices and teach them to be responsible in the process. Some of my colleagues have told me I should 'get with the program'. After all, they say, kids need to learn how to make decisions about the use of technology in the real world — and we should be 'trusting' them to make good decisions about their device use. When I have pointed out research to my colleagues saying that children who use less social media are, in fact, happier compared to their friends who use social media frequently, I have been met with equivocation.

I have reflected long and hard on the view that we need to help our children to be responsible users of technology (as if they are free agents and it's a rite of passage for them to be on social apps). However, I don't buy this democratic version of tech use any more — at least not as far as children under thirteen are concerned. Here's the problem: what if there are two worlds going on? One is a 'parallel' world and the other is the 'real' world? In the parallel world, device usage is normalized and seen as a benign and necessary part of a child's world. Children need to stay connected so their use of digital devices is held up as a right. Anyone who dares differ from that version of reality is seen as a luddite.

However, in the real world there are some benefits but also some real dangers for children who are not old enough to critique what they are viewing nor understand the effects of what is happening to them. A key inclination of the tween and teenage years is social comparison. But what if what they are seeing are comparisons they can't live up to? What if this constant comparison is with so many beautiful, happy and unrealistic situations that are out of their ability to control? Seeing so many beautiful others, who only want to post themselves looking good, can be risky terrain for your children and tweens. On the worldwide web they are exposed to so many more 'others' where there is not even an eyelash out of place.

Our children need to be educated about the way social media platforms are designed. Addictive design is achieved when algorithms are used by device designers to hook its users in. Here are the facts about the most popular social media platforms and online games your child will soon be or is currently using:

» They are run by profit-making companies, so they want customers to stay on their platform, or continue to play their game, downloading special offers to unlock more levels.

» A key feature of the design of these platforms is a concept called 'stickiness'. The 'stickiness' of a platform is based on addictive design. That is, they are designed to sustain a user's attention and offer actual or perceived rewards for continuing to use the platform.

» Algorithms drive users toward previous-interest web pages, accounts or games. These algorithms are designed to funnel users towards subject material consistent with previous searches and likes.

» The addictive design of social media applications and online games can be stronger than a child's ability to control their use. That's what addictive design is; it aims to drive users towards more use.

Children, by definition, are dependent in nature. In other words, they are more affected by what their parents allow them to see than adults are themselves. The phrase 'tech addicted' is widely misused at present. Still, the reason we need restrictions on children's use of social media apps and online games is to protect children from practices that are not good for them. The dictionary definition of addiction is: 'the fact or condition of being addicted to a particular substance or activity'. For example, 'He committed the offence to finance his drug addiction.'

While it might not be appropriate to label a child as 'addicted' to technology, as they might still be in a developmental stage, we can highlight the way addictive design creates 'habit-forming' behaviours in children. Jenny Radesky, a developmental-behavioural pediatrician and Assistant Professor of Pediatrics at the University of Michigan Medical School, wrote the guidelines for screen times for the American Academy of Pediatrics. She says of addictive design. 'I find that [use of the word 'addicted'] especially problematic when it comes to young kids because young kids have no meta-awareness about when a technology is trying to lure them in.'[4] In addition, she highlights other issues around technology use, such as the impact on a child's sleep habits, development, and development of self-regulation.

If your child is having trouble detaching themselves from a tech application, it could be they are at the beginning of a journey of overuse. Early-stage 'overuse' by your child at the expense of a more balanced life (e.g. socializing with family or having face-to-face time with friends) might be something you can nip in the bud by developing a contract with your child. My colleague Jocelyn Brewer has some good tips about developing a family tech agreement, which you can find at www.digitalnutrition.com.au.

The through-theme here is that you need to monitor what they use and limit the amount of time they use these devices. You also need to talk with them about these things so that you can keep the communication open between what you and your child are seeing on the net. With 40 per cent of children under thirteen using Instagram we would be naive to think that it is not affecting them.[5]

In a recent study by Facebook (the owner of Instagram), its own research showed that one-third of girls who already felt bad about their bodies said Instagram made them feel worse. Both boys and girls say they are affected by being on Instagram — 40 per cent of boy users of Instagram said they experienced negative social comparison.[6] When pushed to back up their claims on the benign nature of Instagram use, Facebook diffused the negative effects of Instagram by saying that teenagers needed to be connected and that social apps, like Instagram, provide a platform for this to occur.

You might well believe that your child is different, but what makes Instagram addictive is that once a child starts looking at certain themes like dieting or body image pages, mathematical algorithms keep throwing up sites and links and images that conform to those searches. That's the long and the short of it. It can be insidious and subtle, but nonetheless a problem for children.

The damaging effects of unbridled social media exposure are particularly concerning for young girls. American researcher Deborah Tannen says that the shunning of young girls by other girls is correlated with increasing rates of self-harm and suicide in ten- to fourteen-year-olds in the United States. The number of teenagers who feel 'left out' of their peer group (which they see on their social media platforms) is at an all-time high.[7]

I suggest that you go onto your child's devices and set them to go offline at 7.30 pm. You can do this by downloading a parental control app of your choice or by going into the parental setting on most smartphones. If you want your family life back at night-time, this is a way to do it.

In the absence of a strong internal locus of control, it's likely that their mental health will suffer if they are given unbridled access. So, to allow your children to use platforms before their time is to allow external events to have an unnecessary, deleterious effect on their mental health. Allowing them into social applications when they're not ready for them will make them unhappy. This is not just my opinion; the research from the provider itself is saying that children are more anxious and sadder as a result of their use of some of the social apps. I can't be any clearer than that. To maintain your child's good mental health, then, you need to establish boundaries around their use of technology, at least when they are young. While your child is under thirteen you have time to develop their internal locus of control.

» Hold off for the purchase of their first smartphone for as long as you can. You won't be able to stop the tidal wave coming at you, but you can buy yourself some time to improve their internal locus of control skillset in the meantime.

» Don't let them use Instagram, TikTok and Snapchat for as long as you can, and definitely not until they are thirteen.

» Talk with your child about how Instagram, TikTok and Snapchat compare them against *unachievable comparisons* that result in children being unhappy. Help them critique the apps and become aware of how social apps can affect their thinking.

Use the time between when they start asking you to get a phone and when you eventually buy it to help them get their L-plates.

While smartphones give children access to fun, photos and being connected, they also give them access to the darker side of human behaviour on the worldwide web. Children are accessing porn earlier — on their smartphones. They are coming across content that is harmful and frightening, including anti-social material such as self-harm and suicide websites, violence and other sites that promote uncivil behaviour — on their smartphones. Children are sharing information about these sites in chat and messaging at school, so word spreads readily with little or no knowledge of it reaching parents.

On the benefit side of the ledger, there are some clear advantages for young people in being connected through social media apps. How else would they get to know about a party for their 'bestie' if it wasn't for their smartphone!

The decision to give a child a smartphone need not be an either/or issue and it needn't be something that parents should merely accede to. Just as children grow towards independence as they mature, it is probably a good idea that they earn the right to have access to a smartphone, over time. After all, I am assuming that you will be paying for it one way or another!

Purchasing a child's first smartphone: five tips

Here are my five tips for parents considering getting a smartphone for their child.

1. **Consider getting a non-smartphone**, before graduating to an eventual purchase of a smartphone.

2. **Keep an eye on their internet use at home first** and talk with them and guide them about their internet

safety. Set up filters on their laptop to keep out the nasties. It's not hard to do this these days.

3. **Don't give them a smartphone or let them have access to social media platforms until they're at least thirteen.** That's the recommendation by the regulators, who say there is an age threshold for Instagram, TikTok and other platforms.

4. **If you end up buying a smartphone before they reach thirteen, keep their phone at home on school days.** They'll survive without their phone at school, and besides, they'll be less distracted so they can learn better.

5. **Develop a smartphone contract with your child.** See Jocelyn Brewer's website for an example of this type of contract. https://jocelynbrewer.com/resources/

Regrets, I've had a few

I expect that what I am about to discuss might be hard for some of you. The pressure to give in to a child's demands for technology use can be significant and the 'keeping up with Joneses' pressure can also be persuasive. However, this is your child, not someone else's. And there is growing evidence that children are becoming more distracted and less able to pay attention — something vital for them to understand complicated ideas and process their emotions. You'll need to keep in mind that your child's mind is not fully developed and they will not be able to keep tabs on too many things at once. They won't always be able to discern what is good for them. If you have already let the genie out of the bottle as far as Instagram is concerned or if you've given them a smartphone too early, you can change your mind and delete or block it. You can give them a non-smartphone if you need to be in touch with them.

I get it. We can't protect our children from the real world forever — and it would be naive of us to assume that they won't be exposed to social media platforms through their friends' phones. That said, we can at least stave off the influence of a network communication system which, when left unfiltered, has been shown to negatively affect young children's mental health. It is our role — as parents and carers — to be diligent with what we hand our children. The time will come for them to have a more liberal use of technology, with all the benefits that brings. In the meantime, our time and efforts are better spent helping our children to develop a strong sense of agency, so that they will be critical of the role that the internet and social apps play in their lives.

It is one thing to say we should give children a licence to use technology and teach them to be responsible in using it; it is quite another thing to assume that they will be able to control its use — especially when Instagram and other platforms use 'addictive design' to keep users hooked in.

Here are some basic rules about tech use:

» Balance your child's time in front of screens with other social activities.

» No technology an hour before they go to bed.

» Talk with your children about their technology use as they may not be as savvy as they seem.

Gaze at your children

With the rise of device usage by parents there has been a decrease in the number of parents who regularly 'look' at their children. Equally, *children* are not looking at their parents as much. The evidence is mounting to confirm our suspicion that devices are interfering with the amount of time parents 'gaze' at their infants and toddlers. Over the past two decades, there has been a reduction in eye-to-eye contact between parents and children. And that creates a bit of a problem. If parents do not take the time to gaze at their infants, infants don't gain the practice they need at getting excited and then being calmed. The excitement-to-soothing dynamic is a foundation for self-regulation. Alan Schore, a renowned infant psychiatrist, says that early eye-gaze from about two months onwards is a necessary condition for the *later* development of self-regulation. This is a relatively big deal. If eye gaze is the basis for eventual greater self-regulation, then it is important that we consciously look at our children each and every day.

A friend of mine, Dr Kate Daniels, who is a highly experienced speech pathologist, says that she is seeing more 'autistic-looking' children, but these children are not autistic. She's merely saying she's seeing more children who cannot hold eye gaze. We have speculated that this might be related to a lack of attachment experiences between adults and children: the decreasing rates of breastfeeding, parents being distracted by their devices and, then, devices being used as babysitting accoutrements.

Quite worryingly, Canadian research has shown that over two hours of screen time per day is associated with a significant rise in behavioural problems in children.[8] The World Health Organization has recently released its guidelines for infant exposure to devices and it recommends children under five should get 'not very much screen time and one-year-old infants, none at all'.[9] Just saying.

Radical downtime

Our bodies and minds are linked, and the part of the brain that tells the body to move is adjacent to the part that is responsible for clear-headed thinking. Exercise does more to help clear-thinking than thinking does on its own. This is, in part, because it stimulates and strengthens the medial prefrontal cortex's control functions. Exercise is also critical to a state of relaxed alertness. By walking, running or swimming we can improve our ability for 'mental processing'. This processing, or going over things, can be an important facet of healthy living.

In Stixrud and Johnson's book, *The Thriving Child*, on how to set up good circumstances for a child's healthy life, they talk about the Buddha Brain, and the way it gets used. The Buddha Brain is a metaphor for a settled brain — the brain in its resting state. Our Buddha Brain kicks into action when we are not doing anything that requires focus. We're not concentrating on any one thing (like being on our devices) and we're wondering about the days ahead or the days that have just gone by.

The default mode network (DMN) is a large-scale network of interacting brain regions known to have activity highly correlated with each other and distinct from other networks in the brain. Stixrud and Johnson say, 'Our understanding of its functioning is still new, but we know it must be very important, as it uses 60 to 80 per cent of the brain's energy.'[10] When we're sitting in a waiting room or unwinding after dinner, if we're not reading, watching television or on the phone, our default mode network is processing our lives. It activates when we daydream, during certain kinds of meditation, and when we lie in bed before going to sleep. This is the system for self-reflection and reflection about others. It is the part of us that goes 'offline'.

A healthy default mode network is necessary for the human brain to:

» store information in more permanent locations
» gain perspective
» process complicated ideas
» be truly creative.

When we replay scenarios excessively, or when doing so is painful and we engage in negative thought loops, that's not healthy mind-wandering — it's ruminating. This is an important distinction.

We all need unstressed periods of downtime every day. Our culture values getting things done. But research shows us just how important it is to have radical downtime as well. The more efficient the DMN is at toggling on and off, the better it becomes at processing life events. People who are efficient at toggling their DMN on and off have better mental health. It's like having an efficient stress response, which turns on quickly when needed and turns off quickly when not needed. In people with anxiety, the DMN does not function efficiently.

We live in a world where downtime often competes with being busy, as if people's lives can be measured by how *little* downtime they have. This hyper-productivity trickles down to our children. It turns out that periods of connection coupled with periods of quiet time are good for us. If there is one thing I hope you will do differently after reading this book, it is to let your children do nothing — or, at the very least, have phone-free times.

A postscript

You may have let some of these issues slide in recent times. Life gets busy — and the busyness of life can mean we can let standards slip. You can't undo what you have and haven't done.

That said, I can't sugar-coat any of this. Your children will need to get these basics bedded down if you're going to make a dent in their anxiety.

They will need 'reminding' and you will need to configure things at home so their mind is kept in good shape. If you want them to learn to manage their anxiety, you need to:

» ensure they are in bed by a certain time — and up at a certain time

» enforce limits on their device usage (until they're teenagers — and even then, apply some rules)

» strive to meaningfully eyeball your children every day

» ensure they get time outside and away from technology by going for a walk or doing repetitive exercise, like swimming.

So, from now on, orient yourself to establish some routines that will underpin their ability to learn how to maintain their mind and manage their anxiety. You don't have to be perfect in each of these areas. But 70 per cent is better than 20 per cent, if you get my drift ...

Summary

» A key ingredient in your child's capacity to handle anxiety is in them having a mind that is well maintained.

» There are four main areas in which you need to have 'the main say': how much sleep your child gets; the extent and the type of technology your child consumes; maintaining a good attachment relationship with your child; and getting radical downtime.

» Even if you are 70 per cent better in these areas (sleep, tech, attachment, radical downtime) that's good enough.

9.

Skill them to tame their fears

It is normal for all of us to experience fear in certain circumstances. Something might happen suddenly — and quickly enough — that our heart jumps and it pumps harder. If you were to step onto the road and a car whizzes past, right in front of you, it is a normal reaction to experience fright. We would experience a surge of adrenaline and our 'fight or flight' system kicks in.

Children can let an initial burst of fear stop them from doing things. You don't want to let them get into this habit without teaching them how to control their fear. If this happens, this fear reaction can lead them to developing an emotional reasoning way of looking at the world. Where an adult might experience some fear and be able to immediately tamp down or override it, children are far more reliant on the significant adults around them to help them modify their fearful reactions. Routinely reacting in an alarmed way can become a habit. First-impact feelings and thoughts in the child can set off a cascade of alarmed responding. As we saw in Part 1, parents can provide early scaffolding to enable a child to return to calm. This is not by reassuring them but rather by facilitating *their* ability to calm themselves down. To do this, children need adults around them who can both support and challenge them to 'have a go'.

Nearly all adults can control their fear

I am a big fan of *Star Trek: Discovery*. In the second episode of Series 3, the spaceship, *Discovery*, crash-lands on an alien planet. The captain (Saru, a Kelpian) and one his staff, Ensign Tilly (a human), set off from their crashed spaceship to find out who else is on the planet. Along the way, Ensign Tilly expresses fear about who they might encounter, and she says to Captain Saru, 'I can't help but fear we may be walking into a trap.' Captain Saru turns to her and says, 'Ensign, I would never expect any of my crew to not have fear. But I would ask you to contain it, now. Are you with me, Ensign?' Ensign Tilly hesitates for a moment but then replies, '100 per cent, Captain!'

Let's talk about Ensign Tilly. We're assuming a few things about her (well, Captain Saru is). First, he is assuming that *Ensign Tilly is afraid*. Second, he is assuming that she *can* 'contain' her fear — that is, she can call on a capacity within herself to modify her fear reaction. Third, he is assuming (maybe) that she knows *how* to do that.

For most adults, of course, his first and second assumptions are correct. Most adults *can* govern their fear or pull themselves into order 'at will'. And most adults have some capacity to 'calm the farm' or to return themselves to *equilibrium*. Good word, huh? Equilibrium is otherwise called our state of rest. It's the level we normally function at and it's where we return to after being alarmed. Our heart rate slows and we feel calmer. Helping your child to return to calm is something you can do — but they will need some help with the 'how' part.

There are a few things to remember about fear:

» Fear is usually a reaction to something that is unexpected or imminent.

» Fear can be associated with a previous situation (e.g. having been bitten by a dog, you'll be more afraid of future encounters with dogs).

» Most fear can be self-calmed in adults.

» Children can be taught ways to *modify* their reactions to stressors.

You'll remember that Captain Saru 'reminded' his Ensign to contain her fear and there was a gap in the conversation ... a silence, just before she self-corrects. She acknowledges what her captain had said and she regains her composure. I imagine Ensign Tilly already had the capacity to wrestle with her fear and to breathe herself 'back to calm'. I also imagine she received training — like many professionals do in high-stress jobs — to calm herself. Sometimes, even for adults, what is missing is a 'key-turn' process by which they can achieve this result. They haven't trained for events like these, which all of us will inevitably encounter, so they lack an ability to emotionally reset themselves. The training I am talking about here is training by which a person can wrestle their beating heart under control by using arousal reduction techniques. Divers learn how to return to calm using certain breathing exercises. And just like divers learn to quickly calm themselves, so, too, anyone can learn the skills to reduce their 'physical panicking'. We just need to know a process for doing this.

To recap. Fear, panic or having frantic reactions are all normal. We all experience fear in certain situations. Let's now look at two processes, or tools, to help your child manage these responses.

Fear management tool 1: exposure

The first way you can help your child manage their fears is to slowly challenge them by exposing them using a 'stepped' approach for facing a feared situation.

First, I want to show you how to set up an exposure ladder. Psychologists used to believe that some forms of anxiety could be 'extinguished'. Nowadays, what appears to be true is that through facing our fears in small doses and by gradually managing increasing levels of fear, it is possible to get all those small successes to add up! What can happen is that we learn better ways to control them. Like other forms of anxiety, a fear reaction usually doesn't go away — but we get better at 'returning to calm'.[1]

This is not the case for 5 per cent of the population, who might experience symptoms associated with post-traumatic stress disorder (PTSD). However, most mentally healthy children can learn self-calming techniques. For the few children with PTSD, their reactions (panicky feelings) are not under their *conscious* control. If a person has a traumatic stress reaction to something, it means that they haven't yet learnt how to control their reactiveness. The therapy for this type of fear reaction is to help the person reintegrate the experience that evoked the trauma in the first place — something called in-vivo exposure. To assess whether this is the right treatment, however, a psychologist needs to do an assessment to rule out contra-indications to PTSD treatment like depression or suicidality. But, again, this is not what I am suggesting you might do. Most children are not suffering from post-traumatic stress disorder (including those children with an anxiety disorder).

Indeed, most children can be taught how to overcome fear by breaking down the fear into smaller, more manageable chunks. Laddering is the main tool psychologists use to solve fear-based problems such as fear of spiders and fear of flying. Exposure therapy optimizes the opportunities for individuals to learn something 'new' about the feared situation at each successive step. By grading a child's exposure to a feared event, the child uses iterative experiences to *disconfirm* inaccurate fearful associations: 'It wasn't as bad as I thought it was going to be.'

The aim is to promote *tolerance* of a feared object or event, the idea being that by setting up a series of successes in facing the feared object, situation or event (including eventually fully facing the previously feared object, situation or event), the person becomes a better manager of their fear. Laddering is meant to activate new neurological pathways for coping or to use 'old pathways' for 'new purposes' — to create new neuronal pathways. 'Feel the fear and do it anyway' is a now-famous line, but it is important! There are times for all of us when we need to do things that we initially feel yucky about doing. For your child to go to school after they've had a bad experience can be a bit daunting if they were to tackle all their fears at once. But the cost of them *not* going to school every time they don't *feel* like going is probably a price you're not willing to pay. Not going to school for long periods of time can really set a child back, as well as be a nuisance if you have to go to work.

Stepped exposure can be used for most feared things. It can be successfully used for helping a child to pat a dog or to 'have a go' at giving a talk to their class. Here is an example for helping a child to play a game of football.

Step	Situation	Fear rating (out of 10)
12.	Playing a whole game	10
11.	Playing half a game	9
10.	Going on the field for 10 minutes	9
9.	Getting gear on and sitting on the bench as reserve	8
8.	Going to the weekend game and sitting with coach on the bench to watch game	7
7.	Helping coach by handing out the jumpers	6
6.	Attending a real game and handing out oranges to players	5
5.	Participating in one practice exercise	4
4.	Watching other kids play in practice game	3
3.	Watching coach explain a technique	3
2.	Having an adult sit with child to watch practice	2
1.	Sitting and watching friends play	2

Completing an exposure ladder for your own situation is easy. You will find a blank copy of a ladder on p. 137. Here's how to get started:

» Identify the desired endpoint (e.g. helping your child to play a whole game of soccer).

» Use a backward series of situations from the most feared step to a least feared step, so that with each step it is slightly more aversive as you move up the rungs of the ladder.

» Commence the program when the anxious child has finally decided upon a first step that is tolerable.

You can 'stage' a child's engagement with something feared by laddering their experience and supporting them along the way (commenting on their ability to handle things or even rewarding their successes at each step they achieve).

In setting up a ladder to help your child face their fears, I'm not dismissing or minimizing that your child will have real fears. However, due to their limited cognitive abilities they won't always have mature ways of seeing things. Peck was right when he said that often what's going on for immature children is that their ability to manage their fears is not always proportional to the objective 'scariness' of an event. Helping a child get back on the horse once they've fallen off can be done if we break down the task into steps, so that the steps are achievable.

You can follow this procedure over a few weeks or even a month. Setting up a laddered approach will require *you* to assume the correct posture:

» Your child is told that you want them to 'have a go' at overcoming their problem and you'll make it easy-peasy for them to face their fear.

» The helper (that's you) works with the child to figure out a good ladder.

» The helper (that's you again) will support the child through an increasingly desirable set of tasks towards a wanted outcome.

» You can set up rewards for achieving success at each rung of the ladder.

Jane and Andrew's use of an exposure ladder

Jane and Andrew found they were at an impasse with Tom not wanting to go to school after the COVID-19 pandemic. Tom had been staying at home for longer and longer periods than anyone had expected. When he finally had to resume school again, he was anxious about how he might cope. You'll remember that Tom already had some misgivings about being judged by others. The pandemic gave him yet another excuse to hide away — to avoid. Jane and Andrew knew that they wanted Tom to socialize again at school and to get back into a proper learning environment.

In the following example the first step, middle step and final step are filled in. If you want to have a play, you can fill in the steps in between them.

Step	Situation	Fear rating (out of 10)
12.	Goes to school without being prompted	10
11.		
10.		
9.		
8.		
7.		
6.	Gets dressed for school and attends one hour in the morning	6
5.		
4.		
3.		
2.		
1.	Gets out of bed and gets in the car for a drive past the school	1

It's important that you celebrate or notice your child's progress as they achieve each step on the ladder. This does two things: it makes the invisible visible by you saying you saw them cope; and it recognizes their bravery, effort and their ability to 'have a go'.

Here's a blank one for you to use in your family.

Step	Situation	Fear rating (out of 10)
12.		
11.		
10.		
9.		
8.		
7.		
6.		
5.		
4.		
3.		
2.		
1.		

Fear management tool 2: arousal reduction techniques

The second set of strategies for helping your child to manage their fear is to use self-calming techniques — which need to be formally taught. For this group of strategies, you need to show your child how to do these *ahead of time*. Your goal is to pre-teach these strategies so that the next time your child is feeling nervous or panicky, they can be prompted to use them. These techniques are broadly known as arousal reduction exercises. And you don't have to be a psychologist to teach these to your children. They're easy.

They can be used when you want to train your child to *immediately* calm down. You know sometimes when you see your child looking heightened or flighty? They might appear flappy or stand on their toes. These exercises are for those types of situations.

The Breath Waltz

If a child tends to panic or becomes heightened, help them to become grounded by asking them to breathe in through their nose for a count of three, then breathe out through their mouth for a count of 'three and a bit' — this should be repeated five times. It's important to breathe out for slightly longer because what's keeping their heart beating fast is its use of oxygen. You can reverse-engineer any heart-beating-too-fast problems by consciously breathing out more than you're breathing in, thereby starving the heart of oxygen. For adults, this technique slows down the heartbeat after ten repetitions, but for children it takes less time. Once they have learnt to do this, you can remind them by saying to them, 'Please do the Breath Waltz; then we can talk.'

Alphabet legs

Ask your child to join you in speaking aloud the letters of the alphabet and, at the same time, tracing each letter on the top of your thigh. Go through all 26 letters from the beginning. By the time you've done all of them, you'll have interrupted the worrying or cycling. So, it's 'A', then 'B', then 'C', etc. — said aloud as you outline each letter on your leg. Say to your child, 'So, when you find yourself worrying and you can't let thoughts go, I want you to do this activity. You can take control of your worrying by doing this exercise.'

Self-safe hypnosis

Teach your child to notice five things they can see (in the surrounding room or space), five things they can hear (in the surrounding room or space) and five things they can touch or feel (e.g. the clothes on their legs or the feeling of their shoe on their foot). Then, do four things they can see, four things they can hear and four things they can touch or feel; then three things; then two things; then one thing. This process should take about 7 minutes to do if you go slowly enough. Say to your child,

'So, when you find yourself ruminating or worrying, I want you to do the "self-safe" activity. It will help you to step away from your thoughts and provide a chance for you to go on ... and to do something else.'

> In the Cooper household, Emma often becomes quickly heightened (at times even hyperventilating). Jane and Andrew were glad that they took the time to teach the three anxiety reduction skills to Emma, who often appeared frantic. By teaching Emma to do this at a time when Emma was not heightened (remember: strike while the iron's cold), they were able to prompt her on future occasions when she appeared heightened and ungrounded. They found that by teaching her these skills, Emma was able to wrestle with her bodily reactions to events.
>
> Some years later, Emma confided in her mother that she was able to use the skills her parents had taught her before she had to give a high school talk. For Jane this was a significant breakthrough. Not only had she been able to prompt Emma to take control of her bodily reactions at various times during her childhood but she had taught Emma a transferrable skill for dealing with a future stress-inducing event.

Summary

» Most adults can calm themselves 'at will' — and quite quickly. Children can be trained to do this.

» It is possible for adults to use their medial pre-frontal cortex to calm their amygdala, but children require more body-centred techniques to do that.

» Any child can be taught easy-to-learn arousal reduction techniques for returning to calm. Then, they can be prompted by adults to use techniques to interrupt their cyclical thinking about past or future events.

10.

Listen to them more

Another important tool to help children learn to regulate their anxious behaviour is emotion coaching. Emotion coaching has been around for decades.[1] This is when another person listens and tunes in to what a child is feeling or experiencing. It can help defuse negative anxious feelings. Your child can be supported to 'return to calm' by your use of listening skills, and reset their anxious state. The added feature of emotion coaching is that you can use this technique to teach your child extra feeling words, which will ultimately improve their ability to wrestle with anxious thoughts.

Emotion coaching plays three important roles in helping a child develop maturity:

» It can be a powerful behaviour management tool to help manage strong anxious emotions your child might have.

» Parents who know how to emotion-coach teach their child a language they otherwise would not learn. Eventually, children learn how to use a 'feeling language' to describe their own emotions.

» It will build your bond with your children and help them feel closer and more trusting of you.

The child's absent mind

Children see events differently from adults. This is not the same as two adults seeing one event differently and where one person gets upset and another does not. Sure, we have varying ways of interpreting the same event, which is why some people experience road rage and some don't. However, the way a child sees the world compared with the way an adult sees the world is not just a matter of comparing apples with apples. Children see things differently because they have fewer prefrontal neurons firing. In some situations, they will feel fear whereas we won't. In some situations, we will see risk and they won't.

There are simply going to be times when we will have to use our fully developed adult brains to make decisions for them. It's on these occasions when emotion coaching can be especially useful. If you can coach your child about their feelings, you can promote their ability to better understand situations. The younger the child, the more reliant they are on us to help them integrate strong feelings. Little children learn from us how to settle strong feelings as they grow older. A child can have great difficulty coming up with the right words to describe their internal feelings, simply because their mind's naming-ability is still developing. It makes sense. At two years of age children know about 200 words. As adults, we know over 30,000 words.2 The more words you have at your disposal, the greater the cognitive complexity you have and the better your mental flexibility. Do you remember Travis, from Chapter 3? His 'feeling' vocabulary was relatively poor. As a result, he hadn't developed his frustration tolerance. So his ability to talk to himself was not trained up. Nevertheless, I formed the opinion that a boy like Travis was trainable.

For exercise, I swim in the ocean. Three times a week I swim with around 40 others just over 1 kilometre (or a little more than half a mile) across the arc of an ocean bay near where I live. Because I breathe on my left side only, I can't always see when a wave is breaking on my right. Most times I try to stay out beyond the break. You don't get hit by waves out there. However, there are some days when I get hit by a rogue wave. This has happened to me a good half a dozen times in as many years. At these times, it can be quite alarming — particularly if the waves are high. When it happens, I've learnt to manage my panic reaction a bit better with each occurrence.

This phenomenon of becoming alarmed in an instant is called emotional hijacking. It happens when we are frightened by something in an immediate sense and we have to then work out what the heck just happened. When this kind of thing happens to me, I first make sure I can get air, I then pop my head up and work out if another wave is coming … Then, I know that the best thing I can do is to swim out further beyond where the waves are breaking. I say to myself, 'I am feeling panicked [I feel my heart pounding] so I need to breathe *properly*.' I understand I am feeling slightly scared and alarmed. Once I recognize how I am feeling, I then remind myself I am a strong swimmer and I will get out of this situation — like I have on other occasions. Ultimately, I am able to tamp down my panic. All of this happens in my brain. While my amygdala is still geared up for survival (it always kicks in first), the part of my mind that makes sense of the threat slowly begins to realize what is going on and comes back online (it always kicks in second). It's as simple as that — and it's the same for adults and children, albeit that children's minds are still working out how to do the second step. Parents can assist that part of their child's 'new' brain by being their child's 'new' brain coach, to help them to settle. Through expressing empathy or compassion for the child, a more mature brain (which has extra feeling words) helps a less mature brain to integrate experiences. Children need the adults in their lives to assist them to interpret events.

I was in a shopping mall recently. I was ascending on the travelator — you know, the ones designed so that you can wheel your shopping cart onto them. As I got to the top, a small boy about four years old was just about to go onto the travelator heading down. He stopped dead in his tracks at the entry to the travelator. His mother was in front of him, with two other children. He was caught between following his mother and his fear of getting onto the travelator. He stood on his toes, tapped his arms and shrieked, 'Mum! Mum!' His mother left the other children, went back and dragged the petrified four-year-old on to the travelator, and away they went. While this was a frightening juncture for the child, clearly it wasn't for the mother!

I can see why this mother didn't have time to calm her child. She had two other children she'd left halfway down the travelator in order to get back to the stranded four-year-old. In this instance, this child had no ability to tamp down his amygdala. He did not have the sense of self to be able to return to calm.

It's on these occasions when emotion coaching can be used, especially when it comes to helping your child to *process* strong feelings. Young children's brains rely on significant adults' brains to help them 'modify' their emotional reactions to events. We learnt this in Siegel's Triangle of Wellbeing (p. 25). At four, this boy needed his mother to help him calm down.

A two-brain theory describes this eloquently. A more organized (adult) brain can greatly assist a less organized (child) brain to find the right labels and the right words to stop the child from letting their feelings hijack their reasoning. With more techniques, words and phrases, anyone can achieve greater mental flexibility — and therefore incur more opportunities to keep things in proportion.

'Name it to tame it'

If you want to help your children through emotion coaching, you'll need to find words to describe what they might be feeling.

In a sense, your statements are your hunches — expressed as guesses — about what you think your child might be experiencing. Yes, they will be guesses and it's okay to make them. Nobody can really understand or be certain about what someone else is feeling. But if your guess is wrong, they will say, for example, 'No I'm not anxious, I'm scared'.

As well as being useful for identifying negative feelings (like anger, frustration, sadness and worry) emotion coaching can be used to help your child when they're experiencing positive feelings such as being able to tune in to when they're happy, excited or proud. Identifying their feelings like this helps them to feel good but also gives them a vehicle to process positive emotion.

An example from the Cooper household

Let me show you how Jane handles an emotion coaching conversation with Emma, just as Emma is preparing to go to bed.

Emma is sneaking her phone with her into her room after Andrew and Jane had previously decided on a no-phones-in-the-bedroom policy at their place. In a 'serve and return' manner, Jane is tailoring her response to have an effect; her aim is to help Emma identify what she is feeling and at the same time to connect Emma's frantic self with her more rational self.

Mum: Emma, as you know, Dad and I think you will sleep better and be more able to learn at school if you don't have your phone in your room overnight. I'd like your phone, please.

Emma: (immediately looking heightened) You can't be serious! You just want to cut me off from my friends!

Mum: (observing Emma becoming visibly upset, she looks at Emma and leans in a bit and uses a slightly deepened voice) Emma, you're right; your friends are important. I can hear how you are feeling hassled by not having contact with them. (she stops and waits)

Emma: It's not right for you to take my phone. No other kids' parents are like you!

Mum: (looks Emma in the eye and lowers her voice again to be a bit more serious) I can see you feel frustrated by my request.

Emma: It's not fair; I hate you (frowns, closes her arms, hiding the phone, and turns away)

Mum: I'm imagining you're feeling pretty upset with me. If I was in your shoes, I might feel that way too.

> **Emma:** Why aren't you like Louise's mum? She's cool with her using her phone at night.
>
> **Mum:** Let me see if I've got this right — I can see that *you* feel it's not fair and you're annoyed with me for wanting you to get a good night's sleep so you can learn better at school.
>
> **Emma:** I can do *that* without you taking my phone!!
>
> **Mum:** So, you think you can concentrate at school, do well in your exams, all with six hours sleep a night? (she waits …)
>
> (Emma protests some more but is running out of puff.)
>
> **Mum:** (holds her hand out for the phone) Phone, please.
>
> **Emma:** It's not fair! (grumps and hands over her phone)

When you're emotion coaching, it's important *not* to ask questions, as you can see in the example above. While it's normal to want to check out your guesses about how someone is feeling, asking questions stops the flow of information. If a child has a bucketload of feelings about something and you ask them if they are feeling 'upset', they have to go inside themselves to check in on what they are experiencing. However, if you make a comment — something like, *I can see you're feeling frustrated about my request,* the child can immediately answer that comment with, *It's not fair. I hate you.* That's what you want. You want them to release that feeling — even if it's a bit insulting to you. Emma can answer her mother, without having to check inside, to determine if it is what she is feeling.

Any parent can take the wind out of a child's emotional sails (in a good way) through the simple procedure of reflective listening. You can't do this all the time (it's too exhausting). However, it's a very good way to help your child shepherd their feelings by 'holding the space' for them while you help them confirm their feelings. That's the basic mechanics of it.

As well as the benefits listed on p. 142, emotion coaching your child also:

» increases their word count (by you demonstrating additional words to them that they might not have access to)

» shows them you can tolerate their pain.

Delivery of emotion coaching

To take our understanding of emotion coaching to a more advanced level, let me tell you some things I have learnt in my career as a psychologist about the *delivery* of emotion coaching, or reflective listening. If you want to be an effective *deliverer* of reflective listening, you'll need to use more than your words.

You'll need to 'physically position' yourself (relative to your child) and deepen your tone of your voice as you're saying the words.

The words part we have already covered:

» **I can hear** you're feeling [hassled] by not having contact with them.

» **I can see** you feel [frustrated] about my request.

» **I'm imagining** you're feeling [upset] with me.

» **Let me see if I've got this right** — I can see that *you* feel [it's not fair] and you're [annoyed] with me.

These beginnings of the sentences above, in bold, are called stem statements. My suggestion is that you memorize the four above. These will be a lifesaver when you need them. If you take a little time to memorize them, you will be able to retrieve them quickly. They will be top-of-mind when you need to use this skill.

SOLER

Listening with your body and listening with your tone are a bit harder to learn. When I was learning counselling skills, I learnt the acronym SOLER. We, then new counsellors, were told about SOLER so that we sat properly when we were in a counselling situation. It stands for: **S**it, **O**pen, **L**ean forward, **E**ye contact and **R**elax. Each letter stands as a reminder to position our body relative to the person in the counselling situation, so that our body position shows we are attending to the person. *Sit* seems pretty straight forward, but actually, it's not. We were taught to sit at 45 degrees to the person or to sit beside them. (People feel a bit affronted if we face them directly, so it's better to be at a slight angle to them.) *Open* means that our posture is, well, open! So, for example, your arms aren't crossed or closed. *L* is for lean forward, and it is probably the most important letter, because leaning in, just a smidge, conveys to the person that you are there with them. It shows you're interested and that you're tuning in to what they are saying. *Eye contact* and *relax* speak for themselves.

Tone

Okay, now let's talk about tone. If when dealing with a utility company or bank, the customer service representative says to me, 'Sir, I completely understand how frustrated you feel about this' (and they say it in a very muted, low-energy way), I have caught myself thinking, 'No you don't! You don't understand at all! You're just parroting back to me *what you think* I want to hear, to placate me.' It's not uncommon for customer service people to sound flat in their tone. It's not their fault, because they're trained to stay flat. But the problem with a non-emotional, flat response is that it can sound patronizing. It lacks what is known as emotional resonance. It would be better if they sounded a little more animated. To be animated, you don't need to sound as angry or as frustrated as the person you're listening to. But you *do* need to sound concerned or slightly earnest. If someone is heightened, it's important that you don't return with a 1 out of

10 tone. It just won't cut it. If they're 7 out of 10 angry, your tone needs to be at least a 5 out of 10 in terms of concern or earnest interest, then a 3 out of 10, then a 2 out of 10. If you start at a 1 out of 10 first up, you've got nowhere to go, if you see what I mean. Do you recall how Jane lowered her voice?

It can be difficult for us to truly understand how someone might be feeling. But it is important that you try to use your whole-self, using the most applicable feeling words and positioning your body (slightly angled to the child and leaning forward) and your tone (by being slightly earnest or concerned) to show them that you're listening.

By putting a bit of grizzle into your voice, even scrunching up your face a bit — combined with a slight lean in — you show you are trying hard to empathize with how they might be feeling. This is a good example of Aristotle's dictum: the whole is greater than the sum of its parts. When you do all three things — listen with your words, listen with your body, and listen with your tone — it's not just better, it will give your child a sense that you are joining with them.

Key principles of emotion coaching

American psychologist John Gottman, who first came up with the idea of emotion coaching, identifies some of the key principles of emotion coaching.

   » Set yourself aside; it's not about you.

» Listen with empathy.

» Help your child label their feelings.

» Set limits while helping your child to problem-solve.

» Finalize by helping your child to solve *their* problem.

The first of these actions is for you to switch into listener mode — it's not about you. Listening with empathy is the second step, which requires you to *observe* your child's emotions without being too affected by their feelings. Observing and commenting on children's emotions can be difficult, especially if we are the target of their negative emotions. 'Listening with empathy' is different from 'listening with sympathy'. To empathize is to try to understand, without rescuing your child. 'To label' means to provide an accurate word to attach to your child's emotion. An accurate label enables the parent to develop a child's emotional vocabulary and enables the parent to talk authentically with the child. A key saying you might need to keep in mind for when you're emotion coaching is '*acknowledgement is not agreement*'. You're not agreeing with them; rather, what you are doing is helping them use the right labels to help them process how they are feeling.

Apart from empathic body language and tone of voice, the words you choose need to accurately sum up your child's feelings. If you do this well, you can enable your child to ride an emotional wave — through experiencing the words that reflect their emotional experience. 'Set limits' means that while you accept and love your child (nothing changes there), you do not necessarily accept their behaviour. Finally, you want to eventually get them into problem-solving mode. This is often missed out in the emotion-coaching strategy.

Improving a child's ability to tolerate ambiguity

In her great book, *You're Not Listening*, Kate Murphy says that when counsellors use cognitive behavioural skills, they help a person to overcome anxious or depressive thinking through *cognitive restructuring*. They are effectively helping them to 'talk to themselves differently'. Generally speaking, an anxious child is less able to come up with alternative explanations for an event, situation or problem compared with their richer-in-language parents. Nevertheless, they can be trained to do this. There are key ways that a child develops better internal discourses for managing their emotional reactions — and you can help them to develop those discourses.

It's through your listening and through your supportive 'hearing' of how they might be feeling that you can help them to develop their 'cognitive complexity'. We want to build up a child's cognitive complexity throughout their childhood, because doing so will reduce their anxiety. It's a case of the more words and phrases they can find (to describe what's going on), the greater their mental flexibility will be and the less anxious they will be. By having more words and more phrases to examine emotional reactions, a child can develop more sophisticated explanations for assessing challenges and, by extension, to integrate experiences.

Cognitive complexity is worth striving for. And it's a project worth involving yourself in. The nineteenth-century English romantic poet John Keats once wrote in a letter that to be a person of achievement one must have negative capability. This, he said, meant being 'capable of being in uncertainties, mysteries, doubts, without any irritable reaching out after fact and reason'. It is this quality — negative capability — that allows good listeners to cope with ideas that are contradictory or not necessarily straightforward.

The more cognitive complexity we develop, the better we are at storing, retrieving, organizing and generating new information, which gives us a greater ability to talk with ourselves differently. You might recall, also, what Joan Rosenberg said about this. In order to develop emotional strength, it's important to help a child 'ride the wave' of their feelings in key moments. By getting them used to riding emotional waves, children learn that they won't 'die' from their emotional experiences and, second, they will be able to wrestle their way through the painful encounters they experience. With a half a dozen or so of these types of experiences under their belt, they should start feeling more capable of working through an anxious episode.

Emotion coaching increases a child's ability to have their feelings acknowledged, but not just that; it also increases their ability to 'hold' a feeling for long enough to learn how to grapple with it. What you can do by emotion coaching your child is to give them the chance to cool off without them prematurely locking down on a conclusion such as 'It was so bad' or 'My friend hates me'.

The 9 out of 10 reaction we see in anxious children's behaviour is partly a developmental matter. But it's also an inability to 'hold off' locking down on a premature reaction. Some children don't yet have their rationalizing software installed and can't hold an emotion for any length of time so that they can do the second step of arguing with their anxious feelings and thoughts. So they usually can't find it in themselves to know how to 'sit with' the discomfort for very long to either ride it out or come to terms with it.

Counsellors use their replies, like those in bold on p. 151, to show the people they are counselling that they are listening. This is not hard. Carl Rogers, a famous psychologist in the field of active listening, said that when someone is given unconditional positive regard — that is, when they are just listened to, without judgment — it provides the person being listened to with an experience of being accepted. What they also experience is an opportunity to explore how they are feeling from different angles, and through different lenses of intensity. You will remember I did this for Travis. It wasn't comfortable for him, but it was important for him and his emotional development for someone to do this for him.

In an anxious moment, your child might have the 'wrong end of the stick' as far as you're concerned. You might feel sorely tempted to correct them. However, my suggestion is that it's better to just listen. The thing is that it might be just as useful for your child if you can help them name what they are feeling.

When a child experiences panic or threat, real or imagined, it's likely their amygdala is reacting, or they are incorrectly processing an ambiguous event as frightening when it wouldn't be for you. They might feel afraid of doing a class talk or startled by something unexpected. Through your supportive listening, you can play a role in helping your child to manage their anxiety.

When our children get upset about something, we can be tempted to respond in various ways. Returning to the example of Jane and Emma on p. 148, Jane could have been tempted to:

» Get mad and shout: 'Give me the phone, Emma!'

» Ask questions: 'Why won't you give me the phone?'

» Dismiss Emma's feelings: 'I don't care what you feel, Emma.'

» Solve the problem prematurely: 'Okay, take your phone, then!

Your child says to you that they are 'frightened' of going to school. You say curiously, 'I can hear you're a bit unsure about going to school today.' You *don't* solve or *fix* the problem, not just yet, anyway. You just reflect what they are saying — and then shush.

Imagining what a child might be experiencing is one of the first steps in emotion coaching. One way to think about what any child might be experiencing is to think of their feelings as occurring in clusters. I call these 'affect clusters'. When I'm working with parents, I use a diamond image to explain how to think about emotions. Diamonds have faces called facets, so think about your child's emotions as being in clusters, similar to the facets on a diamond. The facets are the faces of the diamond to the world. A child's affect cluster can be identified pretty quickly. In the English language there are over 600 words to describe emotions — and most of them are negative. So, trust me, you'll be able to identify your child's affect cluster, to come up with three or four feeling words when you need to.

Most children respond well if their parents reflect their feelings. In Emma's case, she was mainly frustrated that her mother was restricting her use of her phone. By Jane naming what *Jane* thought she might be experiencing, Jane acknowledged what Emma was feeling. She wasn't agreeing with Emma but merely helping her find words to reflect what she was feeling. The feelings she was naming — 'hassled', 'frustrated', 'upset', etc. — were slightly different from one another but also similar.

Problem solving, or mental scaffolding

Over the last few pages, I've emphasized that if your child is anxious it's important to stay focused on their feelings so that they can begin to organize their emotions with your assistance. While it's important to help children identify how they are feeling, it's also important that they are encouraged to use their emotions as a learning opportunity or a way to solve a problem.

Back in our foundational ideas section, Peck said that part of growing up is learning how to keep things in perspective and not disproportionately overreacting to small events. While your child will have strong and 'real' feelings about events that they come across, they might not have a well-routinized way of weighing up the pros and the cons of a situation or of bringing a scientific approach to life's problem-solving moments.

They will need your help to see the big picture and to develop an inner voice that can think things through. Thinking things through takes mental effort. It is something you can facilitate in your child if you have a process for doing so. This process, which can be referred to as mental scaffolding, is important for you to undertake with your child. Cognitive psychologists do this in a therapeutic context; they endeavour to help a child to look at the facts of a matter, to use their rational brain to consider their reactions to events and to help the child reframe and problem-solve alternative explanations for events.

Helping children to problem-solve is an important part of the emotion-coaching process. By doing it with your child, not only will they learn more about how to successfully wrestle with their feelings (with your facilitation) but you will also give your child important blueprint information about the scientific process for looking at problems: what are the facts, what is the data, what alternative guesses can I make about what's happened and what might happen in the future, and what are possible solutions to problems they will face? It is possible to be supportive yet coincidentally help your child develop habits to be a good problem-solver, to be their own second opinion and to manage their own emotional reactions. In the first instance, they will need coaching from you. This type of practice needs to occur consistently across your child's childhood. Deborah Kelemen describes this as akin to learning a new language.[3] It can't be done in piecemeal fashion.

In the next chapter, we will have a closer look at how you can show support for your child and challenge them to become a better emotional problem-solver — which, as I say, is the type of help your child would receive if they went to see a cognitive psychologist for treatment of their anxiety.

Summary

» The more feeling words your child knows, the more cognitive complexity they will be able to apply to solve internal arguments for managing anxiety.

» Parents need to provide extra words to help a child become more nuanced in managing their anxiety.

» Remember, in the first instance the feeling words come from you. Try not to ask questions but rather make pithy statements like, 'I can see you're feeling angry about this'.

11.

Helping your child think more accurately

When I was training to be a psychologist, we learnt cognitive behavioural therapy (or CBT) so that we could work with people who had developed anxiety or depression problems. It was mostly used as a treatment for adults or sometimes teenagers who had developed these types of problems. CBT had the most evidence to support its effectiveness. Back in the day, CBT was mostly being used only *after* someone became ill. Until relatively recently, CBT had not traditionally been used as an early-intervention tool to *stave off* anxiety. In fact, over the past 30 years I have often thought, 'Why are these powerful psychological interventions only provided *after* a person's anxiety has been diagnosed? And why hasn't there been more of this type of treatment available *before* anything even approaching an anxiety or depressive disorder has occurred — especially in children?'

You will remember in Chapter 4 I showed you how poor thinking habits can be easily established, particularly in immature brains, which can be more susceptible to emotionally derived explanations. Without someone intervening in these habits of misguided thinking, children can develop immature narratives in reaction to life's stressors.

As your child's parent, you are in the box seat to help your child develop more improved ways of thinking. You can do this in short, incidental conversations or at other times, such as when they are facing a more difficult dilemma.

You can help your child to reset their narrative structures — how they frame things and how they question their automatic thoughts. It could take some months to teach the new way of assessing thoughts that might have become habits. Once you have taught your child how to think in new ways, the hope is that they will end up applying those skills self-referentially. Remember, it's a bit like learning a new language, wherein they are learning new phrases and new ways of thinking about things. This is necessarily a scientific way of dealing with problems.

Earlier, you'll remember I noted the difference between anxious children and non-anxious children, and that even non-anxious children become *more* anxious than adults. This finding points to two important implications:

1. Children need to be coached in how to change their automatic thoughts and they will need the help of significant adults to help them do that (the short game).

2. Children need consistent opportunities to apply their newfound thinking skills — over and over (the long game).

Once you have learnt a basic toolkit of CBT skills, you can help your child to manage their anxiety. In a parent-led model, an assumption I am making is that you — with your fully adult psychological mind — can help your child to set up new threads for thinking, ones that are more proportional, more accurate, and less catastrophizing.

The early developers of cognitive behavioural techniques showed that anxious thoughts are the result of how we *interpret* events. They drew on Greek philosophers, like Epictetus (from the first century), to show how our interpretations can mislead us. To quote Epictetus: 'What really frightens and dismays us is not external events themselves, but the way in which we think about them. It is not things that disturb us, but our interpretation of their significance.'

In Chapter 1 we established that anxiety, whether it emanates from an amygdala source or from a cognitive source, tends to either improve or worsen over time. When children eventually receive an anxiety disorder diagnosis, it isn't that the diagnosis comes out of the blue. It appears over time. The downside of this view is that some anxiety problems will take some time to fix. So, even when you are doing the right thing, your child's anxiety may lag behind your efforts to fix it.

However, once anxiety has been identified it is possible to remedy it. By being aware of how patterns become established, a parent can 'shift the dial' on their child's anxiety by first identifying it each time they observe it and, second, by coaching a child in order to replace old, distorted narratives with better ways to manage stress. Sports coaches give corrective feedback to the player so that the player uses the right technique. Deborah Kelemen describes the teaching of an alternative scientific process as akin to learning a new language. It can't be achieved in a piecemeal way, but by repeated practice.

Children with mild symptoms of anxiety can really be helped if the 'adults in the room' use a small group of 'modest' reframing techniques to help remedy a child's anxious thinking. Usually, we see anxiety raising its head when children are facing a challenge or there's the threat of some kind of loss. A child's anxiety is most apparent when they are facing a risk of some sort.

Improving resilience by helping children face adverse events

One of my favourite books of the past few years has been the story of how an American woman learnt to play Texas hold 'em poker. The book is called *The Biggest Bluff* and, in it, the author Maria Konnikova describes how she learnt the techniques of playing poker, and then how she focused on practising the game.

Within twelve months she became the reigning world champion! Yes, you heard that right: she knew nothing about playing poker but within twelve months she learnt the game so well that she whooped people who had been playing professional poker their whole adult lives. Poker may or may not be your thing. It's not mine, really. But what this book covered exceptionally well were those things we can control and those things that come down to luck or chance. At one point in the book, when she had a bad loss at the card table, Konnikova tells the story of how she learnt to discipline her thinking about being beaten — her 'bad beats'. She makes the point that the way we look at something — how we frame it with the language we use to describe it to ourselves or others — affects our emotions, our outlook and our mindset.

> " It may seem a small deal, but the words we select — the ones we filter out and the ones we eventually choose to put forward are a mirror to our thinking. Clarity of language is clarity of thought ...'[1]

How we interpret an event for ourselves, and the language we use to do this, can determine whether we have an internal or external locus of control. That's why parents and teachers need to be sensitive to the language children use in describing their 'bad beat' stories. It's 'in' the micro-moments that we need to 'stop the bus' and correct anxious reactions by helping a child to tame their fears, name their emotions or fix faulty thought patterns. This is done not so much by reassuring them or by taking their mind off it as it is by giving them templates for controlling their emotions. Our job is to help them to look for evidence or find ways to think more accurately. For a child behaving anxiously it's the 'how' we are most interested in. They need to know the new process for doing it. Seeing a problem from a different angle means that we have other ways to come to terms with the issue at hand.

Remember, it's a parent's 'incisive attention' at the 'right' moment that will help a child. You can still be empathic, but you can also help them to interrupt habitual ways they have used up to this point in time.

Think short bursts repeated over time

The common thread across CBT techniques is that they are all aimed at restructuring the way the client thinks. The cognitive distortions we spoke of earlier (like emotional reasoning, all or nothing thinking or catastrophizing) can become a child's norm from early on.

From a developmental point of view, children and tweens under thirteen are generally not so great at concentrating on school lessons for hours at a time. Teachers know this. So they usually make lessons shorter than those for teenagers. Primary school teachers also make good use of their incidental conversations with children to scaffold them into different ways of solving 'learning' problems. They often use 'two-minute' conversations to good effect.

The key thing to remember is your orientation relative to your child's anxious moments:

>> Be their coach. Set yourself to the side; it's not about you.

>> Express your love and care for them by helping them to develop their internal locus of control.

>> Try to facilitate in them a preference for being proportional, being accurate and using a wide variety of words and phrases to describe internal states.

You want your child to reduce their rigid-thinking mindset (locking onto a hard 'no'). Soon I will show you four elements that go into a stepped conversation, using SALON, which, to refresh your memory, stands for: **s**elf-check first, **a**cknowledge their feelings, **l**ist what you notice, ask **o**pen-ended questions and **n**ow what? This is the one thing I will give you to memorize that will, over time, make the biggest impact in helping your child strengthen their mind and develop an internal locus of control.

The key issue here is not the length of any one conversation but the orientation and the quality of the ones you have with your child.

You do not have to be a trained psychologist to use the skills I teach you. It is clear that when a parent (acting as lay therapist, of sorts) learns what to focus on, they can make a significant difference to a child's anxiety when they witness their child being anxious.

Because children are at a different developmental stage compared to a parent, we won't be able to use all of the CBT skills that are used in adult therapy. Your child won't be able to access as rational a skillset as an adult. Their minds are still developing, so they lack two main features compared with adults: a certain level of the intellectual engine room capacity that comes with maturity; and a certain level of ego-strength to fend off anxiety. But this doesn't mean we shouldn't start somewhere.

Helping children use their mind's eye

Our approach is going to be more oblique and more exploratory.

In their book *Parent-led CBT for Child Anxiety*, Cathy Creswell and her colleagues say that the latest therapy for child anxiety is not so much to teach children to be better thinkers or self-talkers as much as it is to help them *test their fears by promoting their independence* and improve their ability to 'have a go'. That's a bit of a mouthful. But, essentially, what Creswell and her colleagues are saying is that kids need to have successful *experiences* of coping and be exposed to conversations that both challenge them and provide them with better blueprints for understanding their experiences. They state that the focus these days has moved away from getting children to logically evaluate threatening thoughts: 'Instead, we focus on helping children develop curiosity about possible outcomes in order to encourage them to approach situations that they would otherwise avoid as a way to learn new things about themselves in the situation.'[2]

When children are little, we should begin by helping them to look at situations in different ways and to solve all sorts of problems by being curious about other ways of looking at things, as well as scaffolding their attempts to manage anxiety. To do that, *you* will need to think of alternative ways to frame events.

Let's take Tom Cooper's reluctance to return to school after he had an awkward encounter with one of his friends. In the pattern between Tom and his mother, Tom tends to immediately catastrophize if Jane puts any pressure on him to go to school. He creates a scene, and predictably Jane backs off, allowing Tom to stay home and play on his device all day. As a single event, this situation may not be a problem; the occasional day off is neither here nor there in a child's life. However, in this instance, we are told that this is part of a pattern.

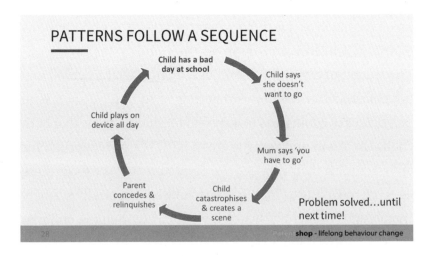

Here's how Jane could have responded. I will call this Jane's SALON action plan.

Self-check

Check in with yourself first and come to a 'full stop'. In this example, Jane asks herself, 'Is now a good time for me to talk to Tom?'

Acknowledge their feelings

If your child is facing a problem or feeling anxious about a future problem, you can facilitate a reframing conversation rather than give them an answer. You might 'know' the answer to the problem they are facing but, in this case, you suspend judgment to help your child to process a situation. You can scaffold his thinking by being curious and helping them consider alternative ways of seeing something.

In this instance, Jane might say, 'So what I am hearing is that you are feeling unsure and hesitant about going back to school after having had a fight with your friend.'

List what you observe

By listing what you have observed about the situation, you will help make the invisible visible.

Once Jane has acknowledged how Tom is feeling, she'll need to shift gears and help Tom objectively observe the problem. In this case, Jane makes the invisible visible by naming what's going on. In this step, your task is to tell or describe what you have observed. Jane might say:

" This is what I noticed and heard you just say: [here, you repeat their exact words to them. By doing this you're making the invisible visible.] You said, you have had an argument with Casey. You told me that he stormed off, and he told you that he wasn't going to be your best friend. When you came home you looked pretty upset that it went down that way. As you came in the door, I could see you were upset, you threw your bag down, and expressed frustration at Casey's unwillingness to be your friend. This has happened a few times now — having spats with your friends. When this kind of thing happens you almost immediately tell me you're not going to school the next day.

Ask open-ended questions

An open question is one that elicits a longer response, therefore encouraging reflection and conversation; the opposite is a closed question, which usually results in a 'yes/no' answer. Consider various solutions to the problem (brainstorm them only); there are usually more than two or three possible solutions (use a yellow sticky notepad to write ideas on). So Jane might say to Tom:

" You're feeling like not going to school. I can see that. Tell me more about that? What's the information you have that tells you Casey will be horrible to you at

172

school or that you won't cope if you go to school? I'm curious, you know. I'm interested to know what went through your mind to suggest that this would be as awful as you're predicting. Lots of people will be mean to us in life; what do you think you'd advise your friend to do, if someone was mean to him?

This kind of 'being curious' lays the foundations for Tom's thinking. Jane is not trying to fix Tom's issue. Instead, she's trying to scaffold the conversation to help him to talk to himself differently. What she is trying to do is stop Tom from prematurely locking down on a hard 'no', which has become his habit.

A caring parent might have been tempted to reassure Tom. But in this case, Jane's going 'behind the scenes' to where Tom's faulty thinking habits lie. Rather than coming up with a demand or a brash rebuff about how his friend had been awful to him, it will be important for Jane (and Andrew) to be supportive of Tom and also to help him to become a better cognitive problem-solver, to help him to develop alternative explanations for assessing events and manage his frustrations — something psychologists call *reframing*.

Helping children learn how to problem-solve is one of the main therapies used by psychologists who treat child anxiety. There are, in fact, whole chapters in books on cognitive behavioural techniques to help children learn how to problem-solve. What's important to know about this strategy is that there is a *process* for learning how to problem-solve. At times, you might have to guide your child in how to approach a problem: coming up with different ideas, working out what to do first, second, third, etc., then working out a plan to fix the problem.

Problems can be of emotional or non-emotional types. Non-emotional problem-solving includes things like baking a cake, working out what to prepare to go on a picnic, or how to draw a butterfly. Non-emotional problem-solving is a good place to start. And then these same skills can be used for solving emotional problems, too.

Following is a list of open-ended questions you could ask your child to help them review their initial (cognitively distorted) ways of thinking. The goal here isn't to reassure the child but to help them break out of the automatic ways they think about adverse events — and to see if they can come up with some new ways of looking at the same or similar problems. These questions are solution-based questions, which are used by family therapists to help a family to think differently. In this instance, they can be used to help your child think again or consider a problem in a different way.

Solutions-based therapy questions for challenging entrenched perceptions

Remember to make sure your questions are open-ended questions, as with these examples.

Indirect relationship question

Context: Your child prematurely locks down on a hard 'no' in the face of a school task and says, 'I can't do that!'

You say: 'I know you admire X [fellow student, sports star, teacher]. If they were here to give you a piece of advice, what advice would they give you?'

Miracle question

Context: Your child begins by immediately using emotional reasoning when faced with a challenging task.

You say: 'If, by some miracle, you were to achieve the task in front of you, what would have to happen between now and then for anyone to achieve that? What would they have to do to get started?'

Exception question

Context: Your child baulks at a task by immediately catastrophizing.

You say: 'Clearly, you've managed this type of situation before when you have been faced with a challenging task; what did you do to get started? Tell me about that.'

Scaling question

Context: Your child thinks in all-or-nothing terms; says they are not going to cope and looks frantic.

You say: 'On a scale of 0 to 10, with 0 being no confidence at all and 10 being very confident, how confident are you about solving this problem? What's the most important thing you will need to do if you were to keep your confidence level 'up' at an 8 or 9?'

If you were to develop one important skill in your child from reading this book, it would be to get your child into the habit of being their own 'second opinion' — and to not accept their initial thoughts at face value.

If you received a crummy health diagnosis, you would possibly seek out a second opinion. So too, you can help your child to question their initial feelings or indeed their faulty thinking. The skill of helping your child to reframe an event and to routinely get things in proportion is not rocket science. However, it does entail you becoming a good motivational interviewer who can provide the right tips and templates for them to develop better resilience-thinking habits.

Psychological hack: distancing

For older children, there is one more technique you can try to engender. In addition to asking open-ended questions, there will be times when you might need to gently guide or coach a child to maximize their ability to objectify their circumstances. This involves helping a child (generally over the age of ten) to get into the habit of 'zooming out' on problems — a technique called *distancing*. This is where someone is supported to take a helicopter view of a problem. I don't know about you, but when I have faced a thorny problem I have often found myself talking to myself in the second person; I say something like this (to myself!): 'You need to take a step back here. You just need to get some perspective on this. Just take one step at a time.' To help your child improve at distancing, you can facilitate their ability by first of all normalizing this type of perspective-taking (by giving them the right scaffolding language for doing it) and by prompting them.

Distancing is a linguistic technique in which you talk to yourself, as if you are another person. Do you remember my friend, Kathie, on p. 61? She talked herself out of a bad mood. As far as your child is concerned, this can be in the form of you asking questions like:

> » If you were your own best friend, what advice would *you* give yourself?

> » If you were to give yourself some advice about something, what might *you* tell yourself?

» This is a situation that many people find themselves in; if this wasn't you but if it was someone else, what advice would *you* give to someone else in your situation?

These types of questions are ways to help a child to zoom out and to consider the proverbial bigger picture.

In this case, you're giving your child a mechanism for stepping away from a problem, to objectify it and to look at it from the perspective of another.

In his book, *Chatter*, Ethan Kross calls these distancing tools 'psychological hacks'.[3] They are ways in which we can use language to take a stance with ourselves, to get a different 'take' on things.

Here's one that *I* have used. I give lots talks to teachers, school leaders and parents. The thing is, I can sometimes get a little nervous beforehand, even though I have been doing this for decades. So, in this type of situation, I will often gee myself up and say to myself, 'Michael, you have addressed hundreds of people at a time. You are well versed in what you are going to say, and you have prepared well; you need to go out there and give your best talk. Nothing short of 9 out of 10 will suffice.' This particular psychological hack is a way of talking to myself that gives me perspective on a problem. It gives me a way to consider a problem as a problem and not some kind of emotional issue to become flustered about. By using my own name, by describing why I should be confident in what I am doing and by talking to myself as if I was an encouraging friend, I gain access to another voice inside of myself to use that can help me build a case for not worrying.

Using psychological hacks is something that can be developed in older children. By using an outside view, our mind can see things more objectively. It (our mind) can consider more possibilities and practise other ways of looking at an emotional issue. However, for it to become a habit, you will need to prompt them once you have introduced it to them. In the first instance, you might have to help your child overcome the weirdness factor, and let them know that a person can really talk to themselves as if they're an encouraging friend. That's why, once you have explained and re-explained how distancing techniques work, you will have to remind or cue your child to keep trying to talk to themselves in the future.

Now what?

At some stage in the conversation, you will need to express confidence in your child's ability, or ask them what the plan's going to be. You might say something like:

> » 'I really think you've got this; I know this challenge is well within your capacity.'
> » 'I've seen you cope with this type of problem before; I think you can do it.'
> » 'I think you have this one in the bag. What's your plan?'

By expressing confidence in their ability, you're helping your child to piggyback on your expression of *their ability* to work things out. You can coach them to use their internal locus of control skills. A lot of what we see in anxious children is that they have lost their verve or confidence, their willingness to 'have a go'. This is a vicious cycle for children to get into. The more they are helped to avoid or the more they are rescued so they don't experience any stress, the more they don't get the experiences under their belt to have a go. This can create a negative loop where their emotional self is more powerful than their cognitive self. I have seen this becoming quite pronounced where teenagers set up sympathy networks if they are facing a problem. If their friend is in any way unsympathetic and tries to help them to be objective, they can sometimes tell their friend that they don't understand them. It's a downward spiral for many tweens who get into sympathy circles and will not tolerate a friend being more rational.

You can help them be more proportional and to be more accurate about emotional matters. You can request of them that they think in terms of percentages and come up with alternative ways of describing things to themselves. You can mentor them to think through the pros and cons of a situation and to resist habitually locking down on a position (e.g. 'I'm so dumb') without first questioning that initial thought.

It's your job to orient yourself — perhaps over several months — to retrain your child's brain so that they can manage their anxiety. But remember, this is a skill that can be learnt. What did the sports coach do? She taught the micro-skills (how to kick the ball, head the ball, etc.) and then she helped the child to practise the skills, *over time.* To help your child get better at wrestling with their anxiety, you will need to play the long game. The three big aspects of CBT are well within a child's grasp:

reframing, problem-solving and learning arousal reduction skills to help them manage their fear reactions. I tell people that a change in the child's anxious behaviour is what is known as a 'lag' indicator. It could take months for the child to respond differently — but as it says in the shampoo advertisement, you might not see a difference immediately but you will see one; it might just take a while.

Final tips

For 'emotional' problems, the main thing to remember is that your role is a *facilitating* one — not a fixing one.

> » Try not to offer your advice too early.

> » You can empathize up front by using emotion coaching (see p. 142).

> » After you've done that, your main emphasis needs to be on helping them with SALON for problem-solving (see p. 171).

Situation, Behaviour, Impact

While we're on the matter of what you can say to help your child reduce their anxiety — and develop resilience — I want to show you a technique you can use at a moment's notice to confirm what I call their 'resilience virtues'. There are lots of virtues we would want to see in our children. Here is a list to get you started:

» bravery

» courage

» perseverance

» diligence

» compassion.

The technique — known as Situation, Behaviour, Impact (or SBI)— is from the book *Radical Candor* by Kim Scott.[4] When you see your child behaving in a way that 'costs' them emotionally in terms of effort, tenacity or perseverance, say what you saw and its impact. The trick is to do this *after* the fact.

Here's an example. You might say to your child, 'In the two weeks before your test [the situation] you went through your schoolwork and studied every night [their behaviour]. I think that effort really showed in your results [the impact].'

It's quite a simple thing — but your child will notice that you have noticed. SBI is a neat way to foster your child's internal resilience.

Here's another example: 'Last night you seemed fairly reluctant to go to Nanna's place for a sleepover [situation] but you got your bag packed and hopped in the car without complaining [behaviour]. You ended up having a good time [impact]'.

A great website that lists the types of intellectual virtues you might want to confirm in your child is https://intellectualvirtues. org/. The founders of this website are educators who note that certain intellectual virtues can be taught to children by adults. These include curiosity, intellectual humility, intellectual autonomy, attentiveness, intellectual carefulness, intellectual thoroughness, open-mindedness, intellectual courage, and intellectual perseverance.

There will be times when you will need to facilitate a child's problem-solving ability. This includes helping children to 'walk though' a problem, acting as their coach. In this case the adult acts to help a child to modify their anxiety. And there will be other times when you will be their direct teacher. In these moments, you will need to show them, train them and suggest ways for them to control their thoughts and be their own second opinion when they are feeling anxious. By teaching your child how to 'zoom out' on a problem you are teaching them a valuable skill they will use well into adulthood.

Summary

» The cortex uses words or imagination to 'describe' events. These words can sometimes misinterpret reality or misrepresent a way of looking at something.

» The process psychologists use to restructure children's thinking is called cognitive restructuring. It is aimed at helping children think more adaptively and ultimately to talk to themselves differently.

» These processes can be used when you observe the early signs of your child speaking or behaving anxiously.

12.

Implementation

Throughout *The Anxiety Coach* we have talked about what you can do to make a difference to your child's experience of anxiety. The evidence is good that each of the main intervention strategies will make a difference. We've learnt key matters along the way:

In **Part 1** we covered:

» Developing an internal locus of control is preferable to developing an external locus of control.

» It is possible to help children develop an internal locus of control and to become resilient.

» Most habits are learnt.

» Anxiety has two main origin points. Knowing from where fear and anxiety emanate helps us to figure out how to manage them.

» There are two modes of strategies for fixing anxiety-related problems: the first is seen in 'serve and return' conversations, and the second involves overtly teaching children how to tame their fears.

In **Part 2** we saw how patterns get set up and how to change them:

» By accommodating a child's anxiety, we are sending them two messages: that they can't handle stress, and that their future encounters with stress will likely be taken care of by someone else.

» We noted how people in emergency services follow a process so that they can keep a lid on their own emotions.

In **Part 3** we looked at five main ways we can intervene to reduce a child's anxiety:

» Make sure they are well rested, place limits on technology and look at them more often.

» Skill them up in ways to tame their fears.

» Listen to them more.

» Help them to think more accurately by asking curious questions and by supporting any child to practice distancing.

» Organize more 'radical downtime'.

Your 'this is what we do now' plan

We know from the research that each of these strategies will individually make a difference, and that collectively they will have a greater effect. To put yourself in the best position to implement what we have discussed in *The Anxiety Coach*, it can help if you have a 'this is what we do now' plan.

There are five areas you'll need to consider:

» *Work out an achievable plan* so that you do 'less of' some things (less reassuring and less accommodating) and 'more of' other things (more picking them up on cognitive distortions in the making and facilitating their ability to 'think again').

» *Work out a couples plan.*

» *Set goals* for your family and your child that are realistic and that you can achieve over the coming months.

» *Communicate your intentions* to your children (including other children in your family for whom anxiety might not be a problem).

» *Use a cheat sheet* to help you to click into action at a moment's notice.

1. Work out an achievable plan

It is not uncommon for any parent to lack confidence in how they are going to actually implement the interventions outlined in *The Anxiety Coach*. And it is not uncommon for parents to face stiff opposition from their child once they begin to accommodate less. The development of a family 'belief' culture is one thing (becoming a 'have a go' family) that will help you; but also, equally important, is telling yourself encouraging things about what you're doing.

If you have a plan, you will know what steps to take. By having a plan you can effectively override the urge or compulsion to rescue your child when you are sorely tempted to. Many people have times when they don't feel like doing things or they are in a bad mood. So, how do we fake it to make it? An answer lies in seeing what other people do when they must override their feelings to do their best job.

Just prior to World War II, pilots began to fly increasingly larger planes. These new planes often had four engines and were a lot more complex than the previous models. Pilots found themselves suddenly having to keep tabs on many factors at the same time so they could keep track of all the things that needed their attention. Some fairly large accidents happened! These crashes signalled the need for a better way of managing all the different elements needed to fly these larger, more complicated planes. To solve the problem, a group of pilots got together and wrote the first checklists. These checklists identified a list of steps a pilot needed to check. Checklists enabled pilots to ensure their safety before they started engines, before attempting to take off, as they became airborne, and when landing the plane. In complex matters like these, they had to ensure that some things were done before others.

Any list of replacement behaviours shows you what to do instead of the old behaviour. It alerts the user about what to do first, second, third, etc. Like many people in high stress occupations, pilots practise a few things over and over. Pilots overlearn what they do. I like to say that, in an emergency, pilots follow a process. By following a process, they keep a lid on their emotions. It helps when pilots are flying a plane — and they're facing an emergency — that they revert to using their rational skillset (a pattern of behaviour they have previously practised, usually in a simulator) so that they can be effective. When *you* are 'in role' — and it is a role (as your child's coach) — you may have to think like a pilot, remembering what you need to do at a particular moment.

What you're doing for your child is facilitating their ability to deal with anxious thoughts or behaviour. It's not personal, even though it can feel like it is.

When you are dealing with your child's anxiety instead of defaulting to jumping in to fix the problem or relieve their pain, you will have to put a lid on your own emotion to do the job at hand. (I know this is easier said than done.) If you want to make a difference to your child's anxiety, it's important that you're proactive in making this happen. This means you shouldn't shy away from your role as your child's coach. You should make it your business, in fact, to 'butt in' on your child's anxiety to help them to manage their anxious thoughts and fears. So, my first suggestion is that you 'steel' yourself. Take a stance. You are not an imposter. You are your child's first teacher. I get it; it's not always easy to know how to manage problems such as a child's anxiety. But at least part of the issue is in you summoning up the courage to get in there and 'have a go' yourself. When your child behaves in an anxious manner, stick with the plan. Some things you should do less of and some things you should do more of.

Throughout the book we have looked at the Cooper children to see how their parents normally responded to them. We have looked at both their normal responses (and why they would have acted this way) and what their child learnt by doing things like this. In the following table, I have listed how the Cooper parents can now act in light of what they have learnt in this book. I call these actions their 'instead' actions. I have listed the fifth column of the cheat sheet for you. It's completed now — and can I suggest that you read it, copy and laminate this for your refrigerator door?

Signs of anxious behaviour	What the child says or does	What parents might normally do
Emma 'feels' distressed in her body and becomes fretful, frantic or volatile.	'I can't do that! No, no I can't just "feel" this way.' (She reels from the event/situation.)	Jane placates, distracts or gives in to Emma. Becomes exasperated.
Tom pesters his mother to ensure she's going to 'be there'.	Tom keeps asking, 'Are you sure you'll be there?'	Jane keeps reassuring Tom, saying, 'Yes, I'll be there.'
Emma invites Jane to do her school project.	Emma says, 'Can you do it for me?' (When Jane doesn't, Emma gets more upset.)	Jane might normally jump in to fix things. She doesn't want to risk a drama and ends up doing the task for Emma.
Tom 'avoids' friendship problems by not going to school.	Tom 'locks down' quickly on a 'no'. He forms a habit of catastrophizing.	Andrew helps Tom avoid a challenging situation by letting him stay home.
Emma doesn't want to go to places or do normal family things. Her bandwidth of 'normal' narrows.	Emma avoids participating in normal tasks. She wants her parents to agree not to do certain things.	Jane and Andrew 'accommodate' by changing a family routine e.g. not eating out at restaurants.

What the child learns from the parents' reaction	Teach the child a coping micro-skill instead
Emma learns that losing control of her body (hyperventilating) is acceptable.	Pre-teach Emma 'return to calm' techniques. Then prompt, and expect that she will use these self-calming techniques.
Tom learns that his distress will be smoothed over by someone else's reassurance.	Empathise with (support) Tom. Then tell him, 'Feelings are information. This is a problem and you can solve it. Let's have a go, shall we?' (Challenge him.)
Emma learns that 'small' problems cannot be managed by herself.	Less certainty, more enquiry. Scaffold her to complete a task by working through its steps.
Tom learns that challenging tasks are to be avoided.	Say, 'Our family has a "have a go" culture.' You need to be accurate and proportional.
Emma learns that her emotional distress is stronger than she is able to control.	Jane and Andrew can't control what Emma does, but they can control what they do. Set up an exposure ladder to help Emma disconfirm her fear of going out.

2. Work out a couples plan

If you have a partner it will be important for you to have a joint policy as far as how you manage your child's anxiety. Otherwise, you might find yourselves pulling in different directions. In my experience, it's not unusual for couples to have differing views about how to manage a child's anxiety. And it's not that unusual for couples to become polarized in how they respond. Once a 'couple pattern' gets established the main responses are typically for one parent to tend to 'give in' to a child's anxious behaviour and for the other parent to be firmer in what they want. Then the spouse who's more lenient will take issue with the other spouse for being overly harsh. It also is common for the firmer spouse to see their partner as being too soft. You need to work this out (away from your child) and come up with a shared plan, which you will stick to — and on which you will back each other up in front of your child.

Once you have worked out how you will jointly attend to your child's anxiety, you will need to watch and wait while one of you helps your child manage their anxiety. A first step to help you work out your joint policy is to agree on your goal: 'To help our child become less anxious and for them to function independently' is not a bad start. And if you can agree on this outcome, then you need to work out a 'this is what we do now' approach that fits with that goal. You can still be supportive of your child but your approach must be laced with ways to support them to manage their anxiety. You don't have to 'give away' your personal style. However, you're better off being 70 per cent in agreement with your partner compared with being in 20 per cent agreement. Once you have recognized the old pattern between yourself and your partner, your task is to not repeat it. Your child might 'look' uncomfortable, and even appeal to you with a pining, sad-dog-eyed look — but you should not react. While your partner is supporting them through a tough, anxious moment (using a method you have already agreed you will follow through on), you just sit there — and don't buy in.

In general, I suggest you put a few basic couple rules in place.

» Agree on your main goal: to help your child become less anxious and function better.

» Work out together what your 'this is what we do now' process will be, and agree on it.

» By all means acknowledge, validate and support.

» Agree to reassure less, reduce any 'aiding and abetting' of avoidance and to not jump in to fix things.

» Express more of a 'you can handle this' approach by saying, for example, 'I'm confident in your ability to work this out.'

» Where possible, scaffold their ability to successfully handle emotional problems.

» When in doubt, back each other up. Even 70 per cent agreement is good enough.

Here's the plan used by Jane and Andrew.

1. Jane and Andrew will not become flustered when Emma becomes flustered. Both of them will withhold their tendency to accede to Emma's demands when Emma gets upset.

2. instead, they will prompt Emma to calm herself using the Breath Waltz (p. 138) technique before they talk with her.

3. Jane and Andrew agree not to reassure Tom every time he seeks reassurance. Rather, they will show support and express confidence in both Emma's and Tom's capacity to solve problems. Specifically, Jane will not answer Tom's repeated questions about whether she will be there on time to pick him up from tutoring.

4. If Tom faces a friendship problem, Jane will not allow him to simply avoid his problems by staying home. She will show support ('I can see that your problem with Max is distressing for you'). But then she will also express confidence in Tom's ability to 'show up' and cope.

5. If Emma seeks her mother's help to make her school projects 'perfect', Jane will not relieve Emma's nervousness at the time. She will, however, acknowledge her wish to do well but will then express confidence in Emma's ability to perform competently, even if her effort is only 70 per cent perfect.

6. Jane and Andrew agree to not give in to their children's wishes to avoid difficult tasks when either of them

catastrophizes. One of them will 'stop the bus' and say 'Let's work this out', as if they are jointly facing a problem, and help Tom or Emma to be more accurate and proportionate.

7. Each of them agrees on a week-by-week 'reduction of accommodation' target. They will systematically choose to do less of some things: less reassuring of Tom, less giving in to Emma's heightened reactiveness, less letting Tom stay home to avoid his problems.

When your child is behaving anxiously, it can be hard to not want to make their anxiety go away. But you're not going to take shortcuts any more. While it can be compelling to want to reassure, help them to avoid or accommodate, remember too, that your job here is to *prepare the child for the road and not the road for the child*. In other words, you will have to manage yourself and you will have to support them to face their anxiety.

To overcome your own feelings of doubt in being your child's anxiety coach you might need to 'gee' yourself up by repeating these sayings:

- » 'I need to follow the plan.'
- » 'My child's mind is not fully developed. I have a 25-year head-start on them in the game of life. I need to trust that.'
- » 'It's a parent's job to direct, train, coach and mentor their child. It just is — and I'm not being an imposter.'
- » 'They're looking to me to be the grown-up here.'

» 'Even other adults distort reality; I don't want my child to become like them. I just don't.'

» 'By intervening like this, I am establishing good thinking habits at a young age that will set them up for life!'

Consider also telling yourself: 'I need to set some goals and follow through on them. I need to follow my process and use SALON at the right times. I need to tell my child how to think in more objective ways how to distance and how to zoom out.' Think, at other times, 'I should not accommodate or over-reassure or jump in to fix things. If I don't jump in, that doesn't mean that I am mean or that I am a bad parent.'

3. Set goals

Large companies often set up their company goals using a SMART goal format. A SMART goal is **s**pecific, **m**easurable, **a**ttainable, **r**ealistic and **t**imely.

We're going to use this process to establish some goals for you and your family to strive for, after you have completed this book. SMART goals can be applied to each of the areas we have been talking about: Going back, let's review our four-point model:

1. Make sure your child is well rested and that there are limits on technology.

2. Skill them to tame their fears.

3. Listen to them more.

4. Help them to think more accurately.

The following table gives a few examples in each of these four areas.

Mind maintenance	From tonight, my child will be off their devices by 7 p.m.; we will get ready for bed at 7.30 p.m. — brush teeth, toilet and read a bedtime story.
Skill them to tame their fears	I will teach them three ways to calm themselves using the arousal reduction techniques from the book. In the future if I see them becoming stressed, I will prompt them to do the Breath Waltz to calm themselves.
Listen to them more	During the next three weeks, I will really try to be my child's emotion coach. I will not reassure but I will, instead, listen to my child — using reflective statements and feeling words — when it is a good opportunity to use emotion coaching.
Help them to think more accurately	Over the coming month, I will try to *notice* more cognitive distortions. I will make it my business to expect my child to use accurate words and more proportional responses when they face an adversity. I will assume a 'less certainty, more curious' position.

Here's what I suggest *you* do. I have left the following table blank for you to set your family goals. Write your own — and stick them up on your fridge. Remember what we said earlier? Any one of these will work. In combination, we would correctly guess that they will work even better. The key aim of this type of goalsetting is to be as specific as you can. It's better that you set a goal to go on a neighbourhood walk with the kids and the dog on Monday, Wednesday and Friday than to say you'll try to walk the dog a bit more.

Mind maintenance	
Skill them to tame their fears	
Listen to them more	
Help them to think more accurately	

4. Communicate the plan

The clearest and most succinct way for you to tell your children how your family is going to operate in the future is to write your child a letter — and to read that letter aloud to them. I'm hoping you will write this letter after you have finished this book, and then read it to your child. I have some suggestions about what can go in your letter; I'll come to those in a minute.

Therapeutic letters have long been used by family therapists. They're often used *following* a family therapy session, to summarize some key themes for a family (usually written by a family therapist) and to point-to or summarize what a family has covered in therapy, but also to clearly outline a future direction. In this case, the announcement 'letter' I am proposing will communicate to your child how you're going to respond to anxious behaviour. These sorts of letters have additional benefits:

» By reading a letter like this to your children, you're saying as clearly as possible what you and your partner will do from now on.

» A letter represents 'a line in the sand' between what you have done 'in the past' and what you will do 'in the future' — and it represents a quasi-formal commitment by you and your partner about how you're going to manage anxiety in your family.

» Having something written like this helps you stop being nervous when you're talking with your kids about your future plans. You don't have to memorize it; just read it.

You can re-read the letter *to yourself* — as a memory jogger about how you are going to respond the next time you observe your children speaking or acting anxiously.

I want to share with you some ways you can communicate this announcement (and other ongoing messages) to your child. Use this one if it's useful for you. But you can also write your own letter to fit your situation. Here's a letter from Jane and Andrew Cooper to Tom and Emma.

Dear Emma and Tom,

We're very proud of you. You're both wonderful children and we love you very much.

Emma, *we've seen you* often come to us to seek help to make sure you've done your projects well. We've also noticed that you clamp down on a hard 'no' and you won't 'have a go', unless you think you can do something perfectly.

It's become commonplace for you to become heightened and sometimes frantic when things don't go as you expect.

Tom, we've noticed how you tend to retreat from problems you might be having with friends at school. We've seen how you seek reassurance from us to confirm that you're doing the right thing. Last week you checked with me (Mum) six times that I'd pick you up from your tutor.

Emma, *what we have done* when we have seen you acting like this is to tell you how 'good' you are and to reassure you. Tom, what we've reflected on is that we also have tried to smooth the way for you by jumping in to help you with normal but challenging tasks. We've also found ourselves placating you by always responding to your wishes to be reassured that we will show up to pick you up from tutoring.

We *thought we were helping you* by acting this way. *But we've had a rethink.* We've recently learnt more about how to help you when you become fearful or anxious — and from now on, we're going to do things differently.

Emma, *from now on we will support you*, but we won't be jumping in to fix up your projects. If you're feeling unsure, we will sit with you (support you) but we will also work with you to see *if you can sort out problems for yourself.*

Tom, we believe that you have it within you to face up to your friendship problems. So, from now on, *it's your job to go to school.* Dad and I will go to our work and you need to go to yours.

We are making these changes *to help you to get better and be less worried.* It could be hard going for all of us to begin with, but we're sure this is the right path for us to take. And *we're really confident in your ability to manage your anxiety.*

Love, Mum and Dad

5. Use a cheat sheet

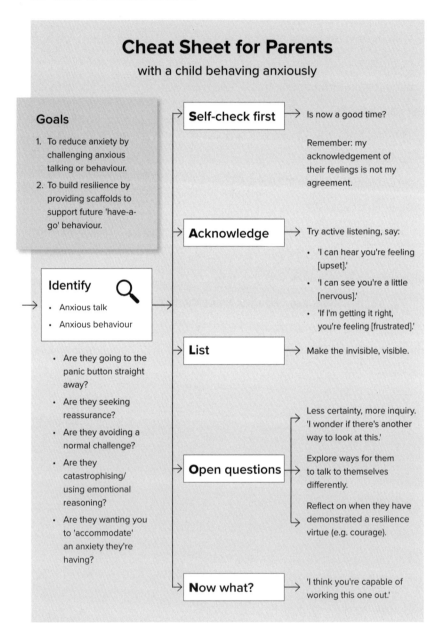

Cheat Sheet for Parents

with a child behaving anxiously

Goals

1. To reduce anxiety by challenging anxious talking or behaviour.
2. To build resilience by providing scaffolds to support future 'have-a-go' behaviour.

Identify 🔍
- Anxious talk
- Anxious behaviour

- Are they going to the panic button straight away?
- Are they seeking reassurance?
- Are they avoiding a normal challenge?
- Are they catastrophising/using emotional reasoning?
- Are they wanting you to 'accommodate' an anxiety they're having?

Self-check first → Is now a good time?

Remember: my acknowledgement of their feelings is not my agreement.

Acknowledge → Try active listening, say:
- 'I can hear you're feeling [upset].'
- 'I can see you're a little [nervous].'
- 'If I'm getting it right, you're feeling [frustrated].'

List → Make the invisible, visible.

Open questions →
Less certainty, more inquiry. 'I wonder if there's another way to look at this.'

Explore ways for them to talk to themselves differently.

Reflect on when they have demonstrated a resilience virtue (e.g. courage).

Now what? → 'I think you're capable of working this one out.'

Summary

» You need to orientate yourself to intervene at the right moments.

» A key way that a child can become resilient is by having a parent who will support them to solve emotional problems.

» Seemingly small, modest changes — repeated over time — can result in significant changes to a child's experience of anxiety.

13.

Conclusion

In Chapter 2, I mentioned how resilience can be constructed. I noted how the Harvard Center on the Developing Child has distilled decades of research on what factors influence resilience. It found four factors that go into how children can build resilience:

» A child needs at least one stable, caring and supportive relationship with an important adult in their life.

» Children need to develop age-appropriate *mastery* over their life circumstances. Those who believe they have some measure of control over their lives tend to do better. Simple things like mastering how to make your own bed go a long way towards a feeling of being in control of your life!

» Children need to develop strong executive functioning and self-regulation skills.

» Children will do better if they are part of an affirming faith or cultural tradition.

In the model outlined in this book, I have attempted to show you how it's your general orientation over the medium to long term which will modify your child's anxious behaviour. They will still get anxious from time to time. We all do. But what you will have given them are the right tools to use at the right moment.

As we saw earlier on in the book, it is possible to turn what may have started as an external locus of control orientation into an internal one. Your children will have limitations in how much they can talk to themselves differently. However, that doesn't mean we shouldn't start somewhere. To graduate to optimally using their own self-talk will take them until their adult years. But with each layer of you helping to construct their resilience skills, you will see some early signs of them developing a resilient mindset. Remember that the brain grows from the back to the front; that means that optimal cognitive control will be the last structure to be built, as they move along the developmental pathway.

When they are small (under five years old), they will feel fear more and not yet have the words to express themselves. Their fear responses might inhibit their ability to think or speak clearly about their anxiety. When they are over five, they might have many automatic thoughts but not be able to control them. In middle childhood, they will need to learn to explore and to entertain other ways of thinking, and how to reframe their thoughts.

Towards later childhood they will get even better at letting go of immediate thoughts, at distancing or thinking again and coming up with alternative explanations. Psychological hacks, such as getting them into the habit of talking to themselves in the second person, can give them a way out of learnt helplessness. They can challenge themselves to do better.

In their teenage years, they will get better at this — talking back to their thoughts or refuting their inaccurate assessments of events. This is achieved with both teenage development and with tutoring from others. However, this ability is also often latent in children and waiting for an adult to instruct or teach them how to use it more regularly. If you can show your support by being empathic on the one hand while also helping your child to become a good citizen-scientist (by scaffolding their observation, evidence-collection and alternative explanation skills), this will help them to develop their internal locus of control skills.

If they're lucky, they will eventually develop the skill of being 'argumentative' with their automatic thoughts. The ability to talk to oneself (in the second person) is a key skill which many adults don't acquire. But you can teach your child this skill. Over a lifetime, we can develop increasingly sophisticated ways of talking to ourselves and weighing up our anxious thoughts and feelings. We can help them to become the boss of their anxiety.

Children are reliant on the coaches, trainers and guides in their lives to help them develop the ability to gain perspective. To develop an internal locus of control, they need people around them to take the risk of placing their child in uncomfortable situations and 'holding the space' for them while they wrestle with strong emotions. You don't have to solve all their problems, and it will do more harm than good if you do. As I have said several times (but it is worth repeating), you can still be supportive even by touching your child's shoulder or arm while you are talking things through with them, and you can also teach them a scientific, logical way of looking at problems. It is not an either/or issue, being soft-empathic or hard-rational.

Do you remember way back in the introduction we talked about how, in using a parent-led model, it is possible for you to coach and show a child how to manage their anxiety? I hope that you can see by now this is entirely achievable by most parents on most occasions when a child becomes anxious. By routinely responding to your child in a supportive way yet also helping them to get better at managing their disproportionate thinking, you can help them to develop narrative structures that are more adaptive and which will help them to cope.

One would hope that if the skills for returning to calm are taught early, you won't have to intervene so much later on. As I mentioned at the beginning of the book, imagine if you saw your child using the 'return to calm' skills you had taught them. And imagine they were using those skills, independently of you, without any prompting. Teachers call this a lightbulb moment (in the student) when they see the skill taught to the child and then being used by the child without their prompting; it makes their job very satisfying. I would hope that for you, too.

Finally. We all face anxious moments and periods of time, and we all worry about how things will turn out. In a sense, we get better at not getting totally bowled over by life's challenging events. We can and do go through rough times and then we mostly adapt. This is partly because, as adults, we have perspective.

Much of what I have been talking about in *The Anxiety Coach* has been about your *orientation* towards your child in anxious moments. While techniques are important, it's equally important that you set up a family culture of 'having a go', to use the techniques we have covered in the book. As you would have gleaned throughout the book, it is important for parents to take charge of their child's upbringing. This isn't a 'you'll do as you're told' issue. But rather, you are helping them by supporting them to grow and to develop their independence.

I have drawn your attention to your child not being a little adult. On that note, it is my opinion that any child under thirteen should be insulated from influences and events that are not good for them. While they are children their main focus is to learn at school and, of course, to develop family, friendship and school connections. An important part of a parent's job is to protect a child from high-level burdens that will affect their ability to learn at school. My suggestion is that you keep them from being taxed by matters they don't need to be concerned with or which will overload or confuse them. You need to be circumspect about what conversations you will and won't have around them. At least part of why we have seen a rise in child anxiety is to do with them hearing and seeing too much human misery, which must have an effect on them.

You might think you should not try to over-influence your children's personalities. However, there are larger influences on children than you or me, and these influences are not always good ones: the unfettered use of the internet, the fear-mongering we so often see used in the media, the way some social apps distort what it is to be 'beautiful' and how this social comparison is affecting young people. These are modern-day cultural trends that are affecting our children's and tweens' mental health.

This is your child, not someone else's

There are a group of activities that need special mention, which might not have been on your list of unacceptable activities for children. See how you go with these. Notwithstanding that other people in your parent cohort may have a 'no holds barred' view regarding what they expose their children to, I want to make a case for putting limits on or even banning your child from doing certain activities. As a parent, you can control or limit many of these influences so that they don't affect your child's wellbeing — and I suggest you do.

And, while it would be totally unrealistic to shield our children from the outside influences of social and other media and apps as they grow into teenagers, in my opinion, we need to protect them from the side-effects of these influences *for as long as possible*. While our children are children, we need to stave off the effects of social media behemoths for as long as possible, especially while they are under thirteen. I would urge you to not give your children access to unsupervised use of the internet or Instagram until that time.

Here are three things I would suggest you ban.

Internet usage and movies that are not good for them

Under thirteens should not be on their devices at the expense of their family or social relationships. Instagram is one of the main social apps used by children and young people and it is my view that you should stave off their use of it while they are children. I get it: when children socialize with each other, their connections with one another are often happening with their devices in hand. But we need to know that some apps, like Instagram, are correlated with poorer mental health outcomes in children. Watch the documentary *The Social Dilemma* and you'll see what I mean.

Exposure to news or fashion stories that feed into children's doubts about themselves

Comparison with others will bring enormous problems for children. There are many instances where fear, uncertainty and doubt (collectively known as FUD) are used by marketers to sell products to children and teenagers. We need to help our children be critical of what they watch and who we allow to influence them. There are forces and predators larger than them that will manipulate them. Our job as parents is to help our children understand how both the media and marketers operate so that they can exercise choice.

Repeated exposure to big existential things over which they have little power

We need to be aware that at least some of the rise in children's anxiety has to do with exposing children to issues they can't solve. It would be unrealistic to totally shield our children from every large existential problem we face like climate change, the decline in animal habitats or other perplexing issues to do with identity politics. We would be naive to think that some of the outrage around these topics would not affect them. It almost certainly will. Some studies show that when children are surrounded by lots of anger their amygdala physically enlarges and so they are more easily triggered to be fearful compared to children who are not raised in these angry environments. So it's best to shield them, as much as possible, from issues such as divorce, climate change and extinction politics.

A theme in this book has been that anxiety can occur when we experience stress but also that our response to stress is something over which we have some control. The key message is that most anxiety can be shown the door, without using medication. On the other hand, stressors are always going to be with us, and we need to help our children manage those stressors by providing them with the right tools to do so.

Soon enough two situations will follow as sure as night follows day. Your child will turn into a teenager (with all the celebrations and vicissitudes that the teenage years will bring) and they will naturally want to become more independent of you. A lot of what I have been talking about in this book is how you can facilitate the development of their internal locus of control while they are under thirteen, so that they will be better equipped to handle stressors as they grow up.

Today, more children and tweens than ever before believe that the circumstances of their lives are determining how happy they can be. They say they are the only generation that has been surrounded by social media, which only highlights people looking good or being always positive. These are false beliefs, and they point to an external locus of control orientation.

Some sociologists say that western society is going through a transition from being a dignity culture to a victimhood culture.[1] Where once we would have shrugged off people's slights or differences of opinions (in a dignity culture), we are now likely to be more easily offended. As we move from being a part of a dignity culture to being more of a victimhood culture, more people are seeing themselves as out of control of their lives and seeing themselves as victims of forces beyond their control. When members of society see themselves as being a part of a dignity culture, they don't think like this. They're more likely to shrug off their worries and to work it out amongst themselves.

We have already seen in *The Anxiety Coach* how distorted explanations can set up house in anyone's mind. At times, these are emotionally based intuitions based on misconceptions about one or another situation. Children are particularly susceptible to these misperceptions because they have a more simplistic way of seeing things. This is not because they are stupid, but rather because they have fewer cognitive tools to be flexible with.

Whether a child is experiencing fear or anxiety — and once these familiar (but not necessarily accurate) words, phrases or emotions become nested in a child's mind — they can tend to apply those same labels to the whiff of a similar-looking situation. So, it is not unusual for a child who is afraid of going in lifts (elevators) to also be afraid of candles and to be afraid of going on planes. When they are not helped to manage their anxiety in one situation, this can lead to them generalizing their reaction to other situations, and that reaction can become a default way of dealing with stress.

Cognitive distortions become formed when children repeat certain reactions (usually emotional ones) and accompanying interpretations relative to everyday situations. These reactions can be overly emotional, even fearful ones. Unless children are taught how to think like scientists, they could form fragmented explanations of cause and effect.

The main process by which adults are helped to redress these ill-fitting interpretations is via a process called cognitive *restructuring* (by looking through a new prism and by learning a new language) when we are faced with adversity. It would be better if we didn't have to restructure anything. It would be better if children's narrative structures were set up properly in the first place. In a parent-led model, you can make that happen.

We need to prepare our children for the inevitability that their lives are going to be laced with some worrying. We won't always be around to protect them. So, helping them to manage stresses by giving them real-life opportunities to wrestle with stress while they are with us is an important part of your nurturing of them. It's not an easy thing to do, to see your child being anxious and not jump in to protect them.

I hope I have conveyed to you a sense in which, when it comes to your child's anxious behaviour, you can still be supportive while challenging them. By helping your child be the boss of their anxiety, there are twin outcomes you may not have initially thought of. First, you will help them deal with their anxious reactions in the here and now and, second, you will have been their core psychological fitness trainer. If your child's resilience could be seen or noticed I suspect that it would look like a certain toughness and an ability to recover from setbacks. Our children would see anxiety as just a part of life — and something over which they would have power. They would have developed a new-found confidence in how they handle anxiety. You will have contributed to future-proofing your child, for when you're not there. If you are instrumental in having contributed to this outcome, you should pat yourself on the back. In my mind, that constitutes a job well done.

Acknowledgments

I continue to be an avid reader and I have also learnt much from walking with and speaking with many others. Being a father means I have learnt from my own children — Dominic and Isabelle — and also from my wife, Simone. I have interviewed many children and their parents and they also have contributed to what I have written in this book. I've been fortunate to have made connections with people who refer me to books and research articles and who continue to help me test my assumptions: Rob Steventon, Terry Laidler, Peter Chown, Angharad Candlin, Ruby Otero, Sally Learey, Ann McCabe, Odette Brown and Bill Scholtz. I could not have done my work without the organizational skills and ongoing support of my highly competent staff at Parentshop — notably the inimitable Hayley Cravigan and Caitlin Kirkpatrick. Over the years, I've been privileged and inspired by people who have believed in our mission and who have provided moral and practical encouragement: David Kyd, Jenny Gundersen, Jill Sweatman, Rossi Lyons, Angela James, Michael Nuttall, Michael and Rebecca Lines-Kelly, Stephen Luby, Sue Foley, Karl Gould, Brad Williams, Tom Phelan and the broader Wallington clan.

My brother, David Hawton, has been in my corner when things weren't going so well. Thank you, brother. This book has been built on the shoulders of the anxiety 'fixers' in our community — family education professionals, teachers and scholars, many of whom you will find in the references section. These men and women, some of whom are distinguished scholars, have sought to ease the burden of child anxiety and deserve recognition. To my editor, Karen Gee, and the staff at Exisle who do amazing 'behind the scenes' work, thanks.

Bibliography

Campbell. B. and Manning, J. 2018, *The Rise of Victimhood Culture: Microaggression, safe spaces and the new culture wars*, Palgrave MacMillan, Los Angeles.

Cave, D. 2021, *Into the Rip: How the Australian way of risk made my family stronger, happier and less American*, Scribe, Sydney.

The Center on the Developing Child, Harvard University 2013, *Supportive relationships and active skill-building strengthen the foundations of resilience.*

Creswell, C., Parkinson, M., Thirwall, K. and Willetts, L. 2019, *Parent Led CBT for Child Anxiety: Helping parents help their kids*, Guildford Press, New York.

Goleman, D. 1996, *Emotional Intelligence: Why it can matter more than IQ*, London, Bloomsbury.

Gottman, J. 1998, *Raising an Emotionally Intelligent Child: The heart of parenting*, New York, Simon and Schuster.

Hawton, M. 2017, *Engaging Adolescents: Parenting tough issues with teenagers*, Exisle, Wollombi.

Konnikova, M. 2020, *The Biggest Bluff: How I learned to pay attention, master myself, and win*, 4th Estate, London.

Kross, E. 2021, *Chatter: The voice in our head and how to harness it*, Penguin Random House, London.

Lebowitz, E. 2021, *Breaking Free of Child Anxiety & OCD*, Oxford University Press, New York.

Lebowitz, E. 2019, *Addressing Parental Accommodation When Treating Anxiety in Children*, Oxford University Press, New York.

Lebowitz, E. 2013, *Treating Childhood and Adolescent Anxiety*, Oxford University Press, New York.

Lukianoff, G. and Haidt, J. 2018, *The Coddling of the American Mind: How good intentions and bad ideas are setting up a generation for failure*, Allen Lane, Penguin, London.

Peterson, J.B. 2018, *12 Rules for Life: An antidote to chaos*, Allen Lane, London.

Pittman, C.M. and Karle, E.M. 2015, *Rewire Your Anxious Brain: How to use the neuroscience of fear to end anxiety, panic and worry*, New Harbinger Publications Inc., Oakland, California.

Rosenberg, J.I. 2019, *90 Seconds to a Life you Love: How to turn difficult feelings into rock solid confidence*, Hodder & Stoughton, London.

Scott, K. 2017, *Radical Candor: How to get what you want by saying what you mean*, Pan Books, New York.

Scott Peck, M. 1978, *The Road Less Travelled: A new psychology of love, traditional values and spiritual growth.* New York. Simon and Schuster.

Schore, A. 2013, *Affect Regulation and the Repair of the Self*, W.W. Norton & Company, New York.

Shanker, S. 2016, *Self-reg: How to help your child (and you) break the stress cycle and successfully engage with life*, Yellow Kite Books, London.

Siegel, D. 2014, *Parenting from the Inside Out: How a deeper self-understanding can help you raise children who thrive*, Scribe, Melbourne.

Stixrud, W. and Johnson, N. 2018, *The Thriving Child: the science behind reducing stress and nurturing independence*, Penguin Life, London.

Taleb, N.N. 2012, *Antifragile: Things that gain from disorder*, Penguin, London.

Walker, M. 2018, *Why We Sleep: Unlocking the power of sleep and dreams*, Scribner, New York.

Endnotes

Preface

1. Creswell, C., Parkinson, M., Thirwall, K. and Willetts, L. 2019, *Parent Led CBT for Child Anxiety: Helping parents help their kids*, Guildford Press, New York, p. 61.

2. See Dr Lyn O'Grady, MAPS, *APS INPSYCH* 2017, vol. 39, issue 6, December.

3. Kessler, R.C. Berglund, P. and Demler, O. et al. 2005, 'Lifetime prevalence and age-of-onset distributions of DSM IV disorders' in the National Comorbidity Survey Replication, *Arch Gen Psychiatry*, 62, pp. 593–602.

4. A recent journal article by Thirwall, K., Cooper., P. and Creswell, C. shows that parent-guided CBT has been shown to be an effective treatment for children with similar outcomes to therapist-led outcomes. www.ncbi.nlm.nih.gov/pubmed/27930939.

5. Manassis, K. et. al 2014, 'Types of parental involvement in CBT with anxious youth: A preliminary meta-analysis', *Journal of Consulting and Clinical Psychology*, vol. 82, no. 6, pp. 1163–72.

Chapter 1

1. M. Scott Peck 1978, *The Road Less Travelled: A new psychology of love, traditional values and spiritual growth*, New York. Simon and Schuster. Pp. 64–5.

2. Rotter, J.B. 1966, 'Generalized expectancies for internal versus external control of reinforcement', *Psychological Monographs*, 80(1), pp. 1–28.

3. Twenge, J. 2004, 'It's beyond my control: A cross-temporal meta-analysis of increasing externality of locus of control', *Journal of Personality and Social Psychology*, review 8, no. 3, August.

4. Ahlin, E.M. and Antunes, M.J.L. 2015, 'Locus of control orientation: Parents, peers and place', *J. Youth Adolescence*, 44: pp. 1803–18.

5. Siegel, D. 2010, *Mindsight: Change your brain and your life*, Scribe, Melbourne, p. 11.

Chapter 2

1. 'Developing inner resources is like deepening the keel of a sailboat so that you're more able to deal with the worldly winds — gain and loss, pleasure and pain, praise and blame, fame and slander — without getting tipped over into the reactive mode. Or at least you can recover more quickly.' Rick Hanson, PhD, 2020, *Neurodharma: New science, ancient wisdom, and seven practices of the highest happiness*, Random House Audio.

2. Taleb, N.N. 2012, *Antifragile: Things that gain from disorder*, Penguin, London, p. 59.

3. Harvard Center on the Developing Child, research paper no. 13, p. 5.

Chapter 4

1. Haslam, N. 2016, Concept creep: Psychologies expanding concepts of harm and pathology', *Psychological Inquiry*, 27 (1), 1-17.

2. Seligman, M. 1990, *Learned Optimism*, Random House, Sydney, p. 76.

3. The idea for this story came from the book *Wildhood: The astounding connections between human and animal adolescents* by Kathryn Bowers and Dr Barbara Natterson-Horowitz.

Chapter 5

1. Lukianoff, G. and Haidt, J. 2018, *The Coddling of the American Mind: How good intentions and bad ideas are setting up a generation for failure*, Allen Lane, Penguin, London, p. 29.

Chapter 6

1. The meaning of the term 'accommodation' in this context is *not* used in the same sense as educators talk about adjustments or accommodating student learning. Rather, it refers to how the adults in a child's life make changes to what they might normally do, such as not going out, or through adults acting pre-emptively to avoid a difficult situation.

2. Adelman, C.B. and Lebowitz, E.R. 2012, 'Poor insight in paediatric obsessive-compulsive disorder, developmental considerations, treatment implications, and potential strategies for improving insight', *Journal of Obsessive Compulsive and Related Disorders*, vol. 1, pp. 119–24.

3. Lebowitz, E. 2019, *Addressing Parental Accommodation When Treating Anxiety in Children*, Oxford University Press, New York, p. 23.

4. Peterson, J.B. 2018, *12 Rules for Life: An antidote to chaos*, Allen Lane, London, p. 122.

Chapter 7

1. Omer, H. https://www.haimomer-nvr.com/post/how-to-develop-self-control-strike-the-iron-when-it-is-cold

Chapter 8

1. Alfano, C.A. Ginsburg, G.S. and Kingery, J.N. 2007, 'Sleep in anxiety disorders', *Journal of the American Academy of Child and Adolescent Psychiatry*, vol. 46, pp. 224–32.

2. Howard, J. 2019, 'Exercise, sleep screens: New guidelines for children', CNN Health, 24 April, https://edition.cnn.com/2019/04/24/health/child-recommendations-exercise-sleep-screens-who-study-intl/index.html

3. Haidt, J. 'The dangerous experiment on teen girls', The Atlantic, www. theatlantic.com/ideas/archive/2021/11/facebooks-dangerous-experiment-teen-girls/620767/

4. Radesky, J. www.pbs.org/parents/authors/jenny-radesky-md.

5. Canales, K. 2021, '40% of kids under 13 already use Instagram and some are experiencing abuse and sexual solicitation, a report finds, as the tech giant considers building an Instagram app for kids', Insider, 14 May, https://www.businessinsider.com.au/kids-under-13-use-facebook-instagram-2021-5.

6. Haidt, J. 'The dangerous experiment on teen girls', The Atlantic, www. theatlantic.com/ideas/archive/2021/11/facebooks-dangerous-experiment-teen-girls/620767/

7. Wood Rudulph, H. 2017, 'How women talk: Heather Wood Rudulph interviews Deborah Tannen', Los Angeles Review of Books, 11 October, https://lareviewofbooks.org/article/how-women-talk-heather-wood-rudulph-interviews-deborah-tannen/

8. Screen Time and Children, no. 54; updated February 2020, www.aacap. org/AACAP/Families_and_Youth/Facts_for_Families/FFF-Guide/Children-And-Watching-TV-054.aspx

9. News release, Geneva Reading Time, www.who.int/news/item/24-04-2019-to-grow-up-healthy-children-need-to-sit-less-and-play-more

10. Stixrud, W. and Johnson, N. 2018, *The Thriving Child: The science behind reducing stress and nurturing independence*, Penguin Life, London, pp. 21–2.

Chapter 9

1. 'Extinction learning in Humans: Role of the amygdala and VMPFC', *Neuron*, vol. 43, pp. 897–905; Wolitzky-Taylor, K.B., Orowitz, J.D., Powers M.B. and Telch, M.J. 2004, 'Human emotional brain without sleep: A prefrontal amygdala disconnect', *Current Biology*, vol. 17, pp. 877–8.

Chapter 10

1. Hurrel, K.E., Houwing, F.L. and Hudson, J.L. 2017, 'Parental meta emotion philosophy and emotion coaching in families of children and adolescents with an anxiety disorder', *Journal of Abnormal Child Psychology*, 45 (3), pp. 569–82.

2. Christian, B. and Griffiths, T. 2016, *Algorithms to Live By: The computer science of human decisions*, HarperCollins, London, p 103.

3. Kelemen, D. 2019, 'The magic of mechanism: Explanation-based instruction on counterintuitive concepts in early childhood', *Perspectives on Psychological Science*, April, https://journals.sagepub.com/doi/10.1177/1745691619827011

Chapter 11

1. Konnikova, M. 2020, *The Biggest Bluff: How I learned to pay attention, master myself, and win*, 4th Estate, London, p. 133.

2. Creswell, C., Parkinson, M., Thirwall, K. and Willetts, L. 2017, *Parent Led CBT for Child Anxiety*, Guilford Press, New York, p. 45.

3. Kross, E. 2021, *Chatter: The voice in our head and how to harness it*, Penguin Random House, London, p. 51.

4. Scott, K. 2017, *Radical Candor: How to get what you want by saying what you mean*, Pan Books, New York, p. 137.

Chapter 13

1. Campbell. B. & Manning, J. 2018, *The Rise of Victimhood Culture: Microaggression, safe spaces and the new culture wars*, Palgrave MacMillan, Los Angeles, p. 14.

Index